T0073486

The Patient-Doctor Dynamics

At the Interface/Probing the Boundaries

Founding Editor

Rob Fisher (*Interdisciplinarian Oxford, United Kingdom*)

Advisory Board

VOLUME 114

The titles published in this series are listed at *brill.com/aipb*

The Patient-Doctor Dynamics

*Examining Current Trends in the
Global Healthcare Sector*

Edited by

Jytte Holmqvist

BRILL

RODOPI

LEIDEN | BOSTON

Cover illustration: *Eternity-Buddha in Nirvana* by the artist Xu Zhen. Displayed at the NGV Triennial exhibition, Melbourne 15 December, 2017–15 April, 2018. Photograph: Jytte Holmqvist. Used with permission.

The Library of Congress Cataloging-in-Publication Data is available online at http://catalog.loc.gov
LC record available at http://lccn.loc.gov/2018960520

Typeface for the Latin, Greek, and Cyrillic scripts: "Brill". See and download: brill.com/brill-typeface.

ISSN 1570-7113
ISBN 978-90-04-38655-6 (paperback)
ISBN 978-90-04-38656-3 (e-book)

Illustrations

Figures

Notes on Contributors

Isilda Sueli Andreolli Mira de Assumpção
Nurse, president of the non-governmental organization Healthcare Assistance to Patients with Epilepsy (ASPE), and vice-president of the Brazilian Federation of Epilepsy (Epibrasil).

Peter Bray
is a senior lecturer and programme leader for counselling in the Faculty of Education and Social Work at the University of Auckland in New Zealand. He has recently edited a number of interdisciplinary volumes which reflect his developing interest in the relational characteristics of client work and the transformational aspects of loss and trauma. Currently, his work considers the role that emergent spiritual experiences play in posttraumatic growth and how self-actualisation might positively intersect with concepts of heroic identity.

Emine Gorgul
is an associate professor at Istanbul Technical University-ITU Department of Interior Architecture. She has received her B.Sc. (1999), M.Sc. (2002) and Ph.D. (2013) degrees from ITU on Architecture and Architectural Theory and Criticism. Her master thesis has focused on dismantling the Avant-Garde behavioural tone in Deconstructivism, while she criticizes the transfiguring ontology of space as a becoming and examines the architectural space through a Deleuzian context in her Ph.D. thesis. She was a visiting scholar in DSD-TU Delft, a visiting teacher at Architectural Association-London and invited studio critic in Hong Kong University, and visiting professor at Auburn University-Alabama.

Nilay Unsal Gulmez
received her degree in architecture from the Middle East Technical University-METU in 1997 and completed her graduate studies M. Sc. (2000) and Ph.D. (2008) in Architectural Design at Istanbul Technical University. She joined Bahcesehir University (BAU) in 2005 and currently works as an associate professor at BAU. Her main research interests include ontological aspects of dwelling, housing studies, theory and history of design, gender and space, place-making practices. She is also interested in interdisciplinary potentials of architecture and searches for in-between grounds focusing on social/cultural aspects of dwelling and place-making. Her work has appeared in Woman/Kadin, Megaron, METU-JFA as well as others.

Scott E. Hendrix
is an Associate Professor of History at Carroll University and co-teaches courses on medical humanities alongside Lani Stockwell in the Occupational Therapy Program.

Jytte Holmqvist
holds a doctorate degree in Screen and Media Culture and Literature in Spanish from the University of Melbourne in Australia. Her main research interests are Spanish, Latin American, Catalan and Italian film, which she analyses from a contemporary urban, gender-oriented, postmodern and global perspective. She is particularly fascinated by the cinematic repertoires of Pedro Almodóvar, Ventura Pons, and Pier Paolo Pasolini, and, theoretically, by the brilliant mind of the late Zygmunt Bauman. Dr Holmqvist writes about film and culture for a number of journals, with publications in, e.g., the Italian *Segmento* magazine and *Senses of Cinema*.

Roslyn Jones
has qualifications in medicine and medical administration. Her interest in this topic is based on her past experience in health administration and her current employment involving the representation of a public teaching hospital in medical negligence claims and coronial matters.

Li Hui Ling
MD, vice-president of ASPE, part of the World Health Organization project 'Epilepsy Out of Shadows', board member of Epibrasil, and coordinator of the Proactive Studio at Curitiba, Brazil.

Susana Teixeira Magalhães
is a Researcher at the Institute of Bioethics, Portuguese Catholic University and a Professor at Fernando Pessoa University, Porto, Portugal. Her research interests are Narrative Medicine, Bioethics and Literary Studies.

Davina Marques
is a professor of Portuguese and English at The Federal Institute of Education, Sciences and Technology of São Paulo (IFSP – Campus of Hortolândia). She holds a Ph.D. in Comparative Studies of Literatures in Portuguese (University of São Paulo) and is interested in literature, film, philosophy and education. She is a member of the research group GENAM (The Narrative and Medicine Study Group/USP) and the NEABI (The Center of African-Brazilian and Indigenous Studies/IFSP).

Li Li Min
MD, BBA, Ph.D., Professor at School of Medical Sciences, University of Campinas, Brazil; founding president of ASPE; researcher at the Brazilian Research Institute for Neuroscience and Neurotechnology (BRAINN).

Ayse Imre Ozgen
received her degree in architecture from Istanbul Technical University in 2012, and completed her graduate studies M. Arts 2016 in IMIAD-International Masters in Interior Architecture at Istanbul Technical University which saw her focusing on Community Mental Health Centre's design. She has been a researcher in the nationally funded research on development of design criteria for Community Mental Health Centres in Turkey. Her work and research has been represented in various conferences. She has been a practicing architect since 2013 and lives in İzmir.

Gabriela Salim Spagnol
RN, MSc (full scholarship provided by FAPESP, Grant Number: 2013/26353-7), Ph.D. candidate at School of Medical Sciences, University of Campinas, Brazil; treasurer of ASPE and of the Epibrasil.

Lani R. Stockwell
earned her OTD from Creighton University and is the director of Carroll University's Occupational Therapy program. She has two decades of experience as an Occupational Therapist.

Sônia Aparecida Bortolotto Torezan
graduated in Social Work and has a Master's Degree in Education. She has been a social worker at the Secretary of Social Action and Human Development in Americana (state of São Paulo, Brazil) and a university professor. She has experience in the area of education, with research in the field of social services, youth, violence, government policies, and gerontology.

Jéssica Elias Vicentini
BSc in Psychology, MSc (full scholarship provided by the São Paulo Research Foundation – FAPESP, Grant Number: 2013/23183-3), Ph.D. candidate at School of Medical Sciences, University of Campinas, Brazil.

Introduction: Words from the Editor

This volume of papers is the long-awaited result of written contributions made by participants attending the conference entitled *The Patient – Examining Realities*, 5th Global Conference, held at Mansfield College, Oxford University, England, 14–16 September, 2016. The conference organised by the multi-disciplinary academic forum Inter-disciplinary.net attracted scholars and medical practitioners from across the world and became an intense three-day opportunity for fruitful discussion between professionals representing a number of disciplines: health and medical science, applied science such as occupational therapy, counselling practices, more abstract and spiritual healing practices through symbolic intervention – with, e.g., mandalas opening up an emotional and much needed dialogue between doctor and patient and encouraging patients also to engage in their own healing process – film and media studies, literature, etc.

This book sheds light on research conducted by some of these conference participants – most of them medical professionals and healthcare providers employed by reputable academic institutions and who take a both scientific and practical interest in the healthcare industry and its practices. The book also includes discourses by academics with a more theoretical interest in health and spirituality and the often complex, even problematic, doctor-patient relationship. Research presented in this volume of conference papers is both steeped in cultural traditions and reflective of new trends in certain countries across the globe. Theories, practices and trends highlighted in the book are ultimately universal in that they concern all of us on a global level. We will all at some stage become patients and are already patients, to a greater or lesser extent, throughout our lives. Given this, it feels vital to engage the reader in a discourse which highlights aspects of medical care that need to be brought to the fore and to the public attention, and to – both as readers and writers – also reflect on feelings and concerns expressed by patients themselves. This will hopefully lead to a greater understanding of what it means to be a patient and to increased levels of sympathy and empathy for what patients are going through. In saying this, the volume equally much highlights the role and significance of medical practitioners in times of increased patient rights and of pressing concerns, demands and expectations placed on the healthcare industry, at least in the Western world.

© KONINKLIJKE BRILL NV, LEIDEN, 2019 | DOI:10.1163/9789004386563_002

With contributors from Turkey, Portugal, Brazil, the US, New Zealand and Australia, like the conference that this Brill Publishing volume is based on this book seeks to educate and provide insight while the reader engages in a both professional and academic discourse. Although at first sight the title of the preceding Oxford University conference may appear to primarily highlight the role and situation of the patient at medical institutions and, also, the figure of the patient as portrayed on screen and in literature, in focus is, as highlighted earlier, also the medical practitioner. The book emphasises the need for us to pay greater attention to the healthcare provider from a both theoretical and practical point of view, and to pay credit to their hard work; efforts that sometimes go unnoticed and might even be taken for granted.

The chapters included in this book have, as far as possible, been organised according to discipline and common topics. The discourses and arguments range from the changing relationship between patient and medical professional and the need to review and rethink this interpersonal connection, to specific breathing techniques as a way for an individual to deal with traumatic experiences, practices relating to occupational therapy and which are, in part, interpreted from a Foucauldian lens, patient-oriented approaches in the field of Turkish healthcare; with an increased focus on community mental health centres and a partial move away from more conventional hospital treatments (approaches that are now gaining ground also globally), so called "mandalas of emotion" presented within a Brazilian healthcare context and used as a method for the patient to self-heal, and the plead for a dialogue to be established between patients suffering from epilepsy and the medical professional, as well as between the patient and family members or members of the local community. Through open dialogue the epileptic may be helped in overcoming feelings of shame and guilt. From a narrative perspective, other chapters focus on the patient as represented in both literature and film, and on storytelling as a method of healing. All in all, the chapters seek to inspire and educate. They invite the reader to become aware of medical practices, and present patient narratives steeped in different cultural contexts while the discourses are ultimately globally applicable and relevant to all of us, no matter where we come from or what aspect of health and science attracts our research interest.

This volume opens with Roslyn Jones' chapter "An Unfortunate Loss of Trust" where she importantly elaborates on increased patient expectations in relation to the doctor, and the treatment provided – partly from a legal point of view. This chapter is followed by Lani R. Stockwell's and Scott E. Hendrix's analysis of "Cultural Theory in Occupational Therapy." These Carroll University scholars expand on issues relating to the relationship between patient and medical professional, specifically highlighting therapeutic approaches to self (as well as prejudices towards the patient, particularly as reflected in a specific case study) and, like Jones' preceding chapter, also Stockwell and Hendrix speak of the expectations of patients who often consider themselves "partners" in the healthcare they receive. Stockwell and Hendrix also stress the importance for the medical professional to act with cultural insight towards the patient, in order for proper medical care to be administered and they draw from Foucault in their both practically oriented and theoretical argument.

Operating within a Brazilian healthcare context, Gabriella Salim Spagnol contributes with two chapters to this volume, the first of which is a collaborative effort with Li Hui Ling and Li Li Min, while the second chapter has Jéssica Elias Vicentini, Isilda Sueli, and Andreolli Mira de Assumpção as additional contributors. "Mandalas of Emotions as Add-on Therapy for Self-Healing and Resolution of Internal Conflicts in Cancer Treatment" provides a case study where a patient was treated with mandalas, originating in Chinese traditional medicine, and where these mandalas aided in the patient's partial process of self-healing. Figures are provided to further illustrate what mandalas are and how they work. In the second chapter by Spagnol, et al, epilepsy is the condition focused on and, as indicated in the chapter abstract, if a "Dialogue with Emotions" is used as an approach to help patients deal with shame and fear related to suffering from epilepsy, social and interpersonal stigma may be properly addressed and dealt with and the burden of having to live with epilepsy will be easier to carry until it may be considered less of a burden as the patient addresses their condition and opens up to a much needed dialogue around this issue.

Also from Brazil, Sônia Aparecida Bortolotto Torezan links back to the cancer discourse but draws in part from her personal history as a cancer patient, which makes for a both powerful and intimate discourse where the reader is allowed to share her experiences in the sense that they gain knowledge and understanding and develop feelings of sympathy towards Torezan: the patient and the academic all at once. Rather than mandalas forming a part of what is hopefully a real healing process, Torezan lists acupuncture, yoga, Jin Shin Jyutsu, ayurvedic medicine, nutritional guidance and dietary insights, as well as – first and foremost – a belief in God and in a higher power as a way for the patient to deal with melanoma or skin cancer.

Peter Bray, Senior Lecturer at the School of Counselling, Human Services and Social Work at the University of Auckland in New Zealand, continues in a narrative vein in one of his two chapters included in this volume: "Presenting the Patient: Through a Storytelling, Illness and Medicine Lens." Highlighting the importance of storytelling techniques, in this constructionist-oriented chapter Bray makes reference to a "Storytelling, Illness and Medicine" conference that he himself coordinated in 2016. He specifically draws our attention to patient references amongst the conference participants; references that reflect a need for the individual undergoing treatment to give voice to their experiences, thoughts and feelings, thus sharing "their journeys toward health" and offering "empowering inspirational support to their families, caregivers, and other patients." Bray's subsequent chapter "Beginning to Breathe" stresses the importance of selfcare and suggests methods that trauma patients can use, alongside more conventional ones, to heal gradually, and to also physically process what they have been going through. Specifically, Bray argues that patient integrity is often challenged "by the experience of suffering" and he proceeds by reminding us that an illness impacts on an individual not only personally but also in a political sense when the person's outlook on life is affected by the illness suffered and with that decisions need to be adapted to the current circumstances of non-health. Breathing techniques becomes one way of effectively dealing with trauma as they help the patient "release traumatic experiences" ... "stored in the body over time and located in other areas of the survivor's consciousness, to bring relief ..."

Susana Teixeira Magalhães from the Universidade Católica Portuguesa in Porto is, like Bray, interested in storytelling as a way to heal and for the patient or sufferer to cope with seemingly unbearable situations. Anchoring the argument of her first chapter entitled "Catching Stories: Building a House for Narrative and Communication in Digital Healthcare," in thoughts and theories by Arendt and Ricoeur, Magalhães appropriately compares the novels *The Storyteller*, by Jodi Picoult, and *The Wounded Storyteller*, by Arthur W. Frank. The main focus is on the power of narrative and the interrelated role of memory for someone to find meaning in life even in the most dire of circumstances. Using the Holocaust and Auschwitz as examples, Magalhães argues that memory and remembering allows for the appearance of a "narrative identity and for the restitution of the possibility of moving on to the future"; however far away that future may be and whatever it may look like. Magalhães' second chapter contribution to this volume again draws from Arendt, a quote by whom opens the chapter and the discourse subsequently revolves around Kazuo Ishiguro's *Never Let Me Go* viewed as a study in how to change the human condition (again, there is a clear link to Arendt).

Davina Marques, in turn, effectively combines references to literature with aspects of film studies when she chooses Denis Villeneuve's harrowing yet impactful and hauntingly brilliant 2010 film *Incendies* as a main source in her highly lucid analysis. The film is based on Wadji Mouawad's play from 2003. Tackling this complex screened narrative scene by scene and theme by theme Marques skilfully manages to create an analysis of the film that reads like a poem and is organised according to subheadings and sections revolving around "Silencing," "Singing," "Writing," and "Living as a Patient and Healing." In doing so, Marques enables film and literature to overlap and the result is an in-depth exploration of the work chosen.

Also working within film studies, Jytte Holmqvist takes the reader of her chapter argument to Spain and, more specifically, to Barcelona. As in the case of Marques, the film that forms the basis also for Holmqvist's analysis is inspired by a screenplay. Prolific Catalan filmmaker Ventura Pons directed his slow-moving urban drama *Barcelona (un mapa)* (2007) with the original screenplay *Barcelona, mapa d'ombres* by Lluïsa Cunillé in mind. The result is a contemporary reflection that includes descriptions of Barcelona as a sleek and modern metropolis ultimately viewed as a dystopia for main characters feeling trapped in the postmodern labyrinth that was the transformed Barcelona of the post-Olympic late 1990s. Indeed, including a number of postmodern elements, Pons' film is concerned with topics like urban mapping and gender performativity – aspects of which can be analysed from a patient-oriented perspective – and all the while the film challenges our perception of time and place. Using flashbacks as an effective way to weave together past and present, the viewer moves from black and white to colour and Barcelona is presented through a series of images depicting iconic buildings through which the film converts the viewer into a touristic spectator observing Barcelona as a character in its own right.

This volume closes with an important and timely chapter that elaborates on collaborative research conducted by our Turkish contingent. Introducing mental health as a topic of discussion, Emine Gorgul, Nilay Unsal Gulmez, and Ayse Imre Ozgen present pilot projects carried out at Turkish Community Mental Health Centres (CMHCs). The three Turkish academics draw from quantitative research, partly basing their analysis on interviews conducted with 60 subjects, with the aim of developing "interim design strategies for patient centred healing and caring environments" and creating "first generation design criteria sets for CMHC units." It is argued that there is a direct link between the condition of these community mental health centres, that provide a community-based alternative to hospital-based models, and the "psychology and efficiency of patients."

All in all, it has been a privilege to edit a volume of papers that concern matters relevant to all of us across the board and that reflect current research conducted in science and healthcare globally. It is our hope that this book about physical, mental and spiritual healing will move and inspire and that it will lead to further research endeavours that produce positive outcomes with regard to the indeed very important patient-doctor relationship.

Dr Jytte Holmqvist
Melbourne 6 June, 2018

CHAPTER 1

An Unfortunate Loss of Trust

Roslyn Jones

1 Introduction

While there is not one 'patient' with a consistent set of expectations, any more than there is not one mould of 'health professional', over the period of my thirty-five year working life in health, I have observed a shift in how 'The Patient' is perceived as an entity, how he or she relates to health professionals, and how he/she is provided for within the health system. I explore why this change has occurred, and contextualise the impact of this change in terms of the growth of the medical litigation and complaint industries. This growth, I postulate, signals demise of the fiduciary nature of the relationship between health professionals/health services and the patient and difficulties in being able to satisfy health expectations at a population level.

2 The Expectant Patient

Patient expectations in healthcare have grown commensurate with the medical advances that have made more things possible. These include the scope of investigations, for example in obstetric, radiological and genetic tests; surgical techniques such as stenting, transplants and prostheses; medical advances in early detection and treatment of disease; and life support measures such as ECMO. So we can expect to live longer, to have a strong chance of allaying cancer, we can revascularise our clotted arteries to give our hearts a new lease on life and we can expect not to die in childbirth and have a healthy child as well, even with a delivery at 25 weeks gestation.

A knowledge of these advancements is readily available thanks to the media and particularly search engines that not only provide survival narratives but also provide a way for the public to trawl through a list of possible causes for any symptom that he or she may be experiencing. So, the patient on some levels is more informed, is encouraged to form the belief that western medicine can detect and treat anything that may eventuate and is, at the same time, primed to receive a certain approach to his or her set of symptoms.

© KONINKLIJKE BRILL NV, LEIDEN, 2019 | DOI:10.1163/9789004386563_003

Associated with this growth in what is possible and our expectation that it will be possible for each of us, is the decrease in religious faith in general that shifts from the belief that our lives are in God's hands to a desire to be able to both control our lives and to insure against any misadventure. Technological advances assist in this insurance process with their emphasis on testing and surveillance with detection and screening programmes to diagnose and treat early for the best possible chance of a cure. So the patient now expects and is expected to have an active role in their care and well being, and we have seen the development of apps that can monitor pulse rate, respiration rate and blood pressure, in order to give us control over our bodies.

An increase in patients' expectations goes hand-in-hand with the growth of consumerism. Patients now more openly challenge the authority of doctors, treating the doctor-patient relationship as a commercial contract.[1] There is an expectation of not only getting value for money but also having a voice by which to rate your medical experience according to your expectations. Patients are no longer patient patients but 'consumers' of health care, 'doctor-shopping' for a doctor that 'delivers'. This title promotes a mental image of the voracious sampler of all things medical who rates his or her experience as an individual consumer who matters. And whether expectations have been met to an individual set of criteria is then broadcast across social media.

This is in the context of an ethos of 'individual rights' and 'entitlement', a mentality that demands a set of 'rights', including the guarantee of a perfect birth, a long age and a pain-free existence, and, finally, a right to complain, receive an apology and pursue a financial or legal remedy, should these not eventuate. There is a tendency to expect to be able to find a rating for doctors on the net, giving satisfaction measures and complication rates as part of their rights and to achieve 'empowerment' to make an informed choice. One of the health insurance companies has established a website named *Whitecoat* with the claim that it will be the 'TripAdvisor' of healthcare.[2]

But patients' increased expectations have some negative effects that are not always foreseen. Certainly patients now have the potential to be better informed, but as Dr John Jury, a GP and Sociologist working in Melbourne, points

---

1   James Hughes, "Organization and Information at the Bed-side: the Experience of the Medical Division of Labor University Hospitals' inpatients" (PhD diss., University of Chicago, 1995), Chap. One.
2   Adrian Rollins, "Doctor Rating Website Could Hurt Patients," *Australian Medicine* August 2, 2016 n.p. accessed 2 August 2016, https://ama.com.au/ausmed/doctor-rating-website-could-hurt-patients

out, 'The Google factor is a hungry beast'[3] and if doctors participate in consensus partnership with their patients as they try to rule out all possibilities of a symptom, health costs spiral. So too do the referrals to an ever-increasing list of subspecialists as each specialist runs a full gamete of the tests at his or her disposal prior to referring on to the next subspecialty area.

The risk of this process as Dr Iona Heath, past president of the UK College of General Practitioners, points out, is that patient-anxiety, as well as the possibility of adverse events from the actual tests, spiral as he or she hops on the testing merry-go-round. She makes the observation that, despite an increasing longevity within our populations, and when so much is medically possible, people are obsessing about illness at the expense of not living their lives. The range of investigations at hand is extending rapidly, which has benefits, but as Heath indicates, it takes time to contextualise the clinical significance of positive findings for any new testing discipline.[4] A ready example of this is in the area of genetic testing. As the NSW Ministry of Health Centre for Genetics Education identifies, there are many ethical dilemmas that genetic testing introduces, including the difficult decision of carrying out predictive/presymptomatic testing. This testing is not necessarily decisive, so is limited in reliability, has implications for other family members, and raises the potential for discrimination with respect to employment and insurance.[5]

A further issue is that, while patient satisfaction with their health professional is important, and second opinions are valuable, doctor-shopping encourages GP visits that relate to a single medical presentation, and care that is provided on a limited history, which inevitably results in poor continuity of care. As well, a consumer mentality to healthcare promotes a growth of medical clinics that are owned and run as a business by non-medical entrepreneurs.

And with respect to the rating of doctors on websites, as observed by the Australian Medical Association President Dr Michael Gannon, there are dangers in publishing blunt instruments such as infection rates. The unintended consequences of this is that doctors will be cautious of operating on diabetics, the morbidly obese, or on rural patients in the fear that their statistics will be

---

3 John Jory, "Who's the Boss in the Doctor-Patient Relationship?," *Australian Doctor*, July 7, 2016, n.p., accessed 7 July 2016, http://www.australiandoctor.com.au/smart-practice/in-your-practice/whos-the-boss-in-the-doctor-patient-relationship

4 Iona Heath, Panel discussion, "Is Too Much Testing and Treatment Making Us Sick," Sydney Ideas with co-presentation with the School of Public Health, University of Sydney, 30 May 2016, accessed 7 July 2016, http://sydney.edu.au/sydney_ideas/lectures/2016/too_much_testing_forum.shtml.

5 NSW Health, "Ethical Issues in Human Genetics and Genomics," last modified February 26, 2016, accessed 1 August 2016, http://www.genetics.edu.au

distorted by a public that is unable to distinguish between relative outcomes according to the complexity of cases.[6]

There is a further concern about the relative rights of an individual as opposed to the population-based concerns of providing health care on the basis of need and an assessment of relative priorities. An individual patient's rights are certainly worth preserving and cherishing. They are a measure of a society based on humanity, but there is a danger in preserving these rights irrespective of the load on hospitals and practitioners at the time in question; or on the realisation that staff are human and can make errors; or on the inevitable inability to counteract the disease process in imperfect bodies.

And finally, as observed by Dr Ganesh, an Indian urologist who writes on the patient-doctor relationship and the growth of litigation, the modern communication system based on social networking groups and blogging is 'a pretence of communication with no physical social angle or interface'. He purports that 'We are talking more, writing more, and yet appear to be communicating less'[7] and mourns this loss of meaningful communication and level of trust in a medical system predominated by 'patient demands for disclosure and expectations of a cafeteria approach in diagnosis and management'.[8]

3   Impact on the Health System

These changes in expectation have had significant effects on the health system. Without doubt there are many positive effects, as there is greater patient consultation and improved medical practices that involve an appreciation of the perception of the patient and the patient's experience, especially in the areas of obstetrics and paediatrics. 'Consumers' have a greater say, with representation on hospital boards for example; subtle changes have occurred such as extended visiting hours, husbands being present at their babies' births and allowing parents to stay overnight with their sick children; and minority groups are recognised with an improvement in services that cater to their particular needs. Furthermore, there has been the adoption of rigorous investigative frameworks into clinical practice with a genuine desire to improve systems and decrease morbidity and mortality based not only on medical outcome statistics but patients' complaints and suggestions.

---

6 Adrian Rollins, *Australian Medicine*, n.p.
7 K. Ganesh, "Patient-Doctor Relationship: Changing Perspectives and Medical Litigation," *Indian Journal of Urology* 25.3 (2009): n.p., accessed 30 July 2016, doi:10.4103/0970-1591.56204
8 Ibid.

But while patients' expectations in the ability of medicine to cure and respond to their individual needs have increased, many of the limitations associated with the maintenance of good health, the delivery of a mistake-free
health system, the adverse event-free operation or procedure, and the perfect
birth from the perspective of the parents' preconceptions, exist and will always
exist. So too will the limitations on healthcare expenditure and what is human-
ly possible, both from an individual level and from the standpoint of the larger
healthcare system.

Significantly, from any mismatch between patient expectations and outcome, there is the potential for complaint, medical litigation and demand for
reparation, hallmark signs of a system based on a level of distrust. Certainly
in Australia we have seen a growth in the rates of medical negligence claims
against doctors and hospitals from the 1990s and in the amounts of compensation awarded in courts. The legal tests for deciding negligence has generally shifted to a more patient-based focus away from the previous doctor-based
approach.[9]

In Australia, this increase in litigation forced the largest Australian medical indemnity provider into provisional liquidation and medical practitioners
have been faced with large insurance premiums. The flow-on effect was to ini-
tiate tort law reform and introduce Government assistance measures for the
cover of doctors in public health systems.[10] So in effect, the taxpayer is funding
a large proportion of the sizeable individual medical negligence payments that
are now largely determined through a system of mediation. In addition, we
have had the development of a state-based tribunal system by which unrep-
resented complainants can bring claims for compensation concerning alleged
breeches of privacy, discriminatory behaviour and failure to provide services
that had been paid for. At a hospital level we have seen a growth in the complexity of clinical investigation with firstly quality assurance, then root cause
analysis investigations on top of the previous mortality and morbidity meetings and the medical credentialing process. We have open disclosure, transparency and information release policies in line with State legislation. There are a
number of investigative bodies such as patient quality and clinical governance
units at hospital level, the Health Care Complaints Commission and the Clinical Excellence Commission at a State level, and at a Federal level, the hospital

---

9   Win-Li Toh, Linda Satchwell and Jonathan Cohen, "Medical Indemnity – Who's Got the
       Perfect Cure?," (paper presented to the Institute of Actuaries of Australia at the 12th Acci-
       dent Compensation Seminar, Melbourne, Victoria, November 22–24, 2004), 17-18.
10   Ibid., 18.

accreditation body and AHPRA, the regulation body for health professional registration and investigation into clinical practice.

The health system has responded in other ways as well, as evidenced by the nature and burgeoning of hospital policies that advise patients of their rights and responsibilities and the way to complain if their expectations about any aspect of their care have not been met. The hospital is policy-driven about many particulars of a patient's care and forms assessing risks for patients have multiplied. There are now new categories of staff such as risk management officers, privacy officers, information release officers and legal officers.

Of late an interesting addition is the patient advocate – a person employed by a patient to sit between the doctor and patient so that the patient can be supported and explained to about consultations. Not a language interpreter but a 'health' interpreter who has a private business around establishing a barrier between the doctor and patient from the outset, in order to bring clarity. Yet clarity is not the effect for the health practitioner who is uncertain about the accuracy with which information is 'relayed' to the patient and the reliability of the information received back by this 'interpreter and advocate' after conferring with the patient.

4   Loss of Trust

So there are categories of staff that didn't exist twenty years ago to attend to the multiple tiers of clinical investigation, complaint investigation and litigation management, a cumbersome set of processes that demands enormous administrative maintenance, and health professionals who are stressed by multiple complaint processes. It seems as if battle lines have been drawn between patient and health practitioner, with high expectations for a flawless health service by the patient and stressed clinicians practising defensive medicine for an unappreciative public. As reported by Bourne et al in their study of the effect of complaints on doctors in the UK, doctors reported a sense of powerlessness, emotional distress, and negativity against not only the complainants but also those managing the complaints. The doctors reported practising defensively as a result of the complaints and perceived that few complaints and their investigations resulted in positive outcomes. A commonly expressed concern was that investigations were automatically biased in favour of the complainant and that there was a dearth of policies for the handling of vexatious complainants.[11]

---

11   Tom Bourne, et al., "Doctor's Experiences and Their Perception of the Most Stressful Aspects of Complaints Processes in the UK: an Analysis of Qualitative Survey Data," *BMJ*

Dr Fatimah Lateef, an emergency physician working in Singapore, comments that the increase in patient expectations 'needs to be managed adequately in order to improve outcomes and decrease liability'.[12] This approach is a consistent reaction but it reflects the 'them and us' division, defensive medical practice and adopts the usual 'cure' of the introduction of yet another set of models. Predictably, Lateef turns to the 'patient-centred health care' and 'value-based health care' approaches,[13] which, although have noble aims, largely represent yet another fresh set of catchphrases by which to 'address' this 'problem' of increasing complaints.

In replies to letters of complaint, there is frequently the standard phraseology – 'I am sorry that we did not meet your expectations on this occasion' or words to this effect. Such statements may be read by the more cynical as implying that the complainant's expectations were unreasonable, but even for those less cynical, many read that this is an apology for the sake of apologising. Certainly, it is 'politically correct' to issue an apology, even though the remainder of the reply outlining the substance of the investigation may dispute the complainant's perception of the care that was provided.

Jory has commented on such political correctness in his recent publication in 'Australian Doctor', stating that today, 'doctors suffer from some form of survivor guilt', fearing to assert themselves against domination by a 'populist political correctness'. He warns against undermining the very strong ethos of caring, confidentiality, and dedication that formed the basis of the treating relationship and that consensus medicine as a model can lead to 'uninformed and psychologically intimidating demands'.[14] He goes on to argue that there are certain strong foundations of the doctor-patient relationship: treating patients with dignity, courteousness and consideration; providing information clearly; and adopting a position of maximum transparency. But he emphasises that doctors are professionals and that there is a necessary hierarchy in the doctor-patient relationship that is based on the knowledge, experience and expertise of the health professional.

Disturbingly, a further sign of a 'them and us' mentality is the formulation of policies designed to protect staff against aggressive patients. Of course staff do need to be protected from an aggressive patient or relative, especially

Open 6:e011711 (2016): n.p. accessed 20 July 2016, doi:10.1136/bmjopen-2016-011711.

12   Fatimah Lateef, "Patient Expectations and the Paradigm Shift of Care in 2016," *Journal of Emergencies, Trauma and Shock*, 4.2 (2011): 163, accessed 27 July 2016, doi: 10.4103/0974-2700.82199.

13   Ibid., 165-166.

14   Jory, "Who's the Boss," n.p.

when there is a mental health or drug or alcohol issue. But the current 'Zero Tolerance' to aggression attitude presupposes that calling Security is the only option, when often, raised voices are symptoms of patients or their relatives feeling distressed and anxious, a situation that can be resolved through understanding and explanation.

In addition, the increase in litigation suggests a lack of confidence in the healthcare system, although one must remember that these cases represent only a very small proportion of the total throughput of patients and a minority of those patients experiencing adverse events. And as Toh et al indicate, only a small percentage of adverse medical outcomes are a result of negligence or fault by health practitioners.[15] In Australia, negligence must be proven before compensation is awarded. Nevertheless, it is difficult for clinicians to maintain perspective and not feel under threat in a climate of billboards posted by compensation lawyers that urges anyone who has had a medical adverse event to seek their services. This extends to relatives who are in 'nervous shock' following the death or injury of a loved one.

The media must share some responsibility for the breakdown in trust in healthcare as well, in that the health stories that are reported on are often high in drama and low in accuracy. Further, they rarely engage in rational or sophisticated discussions about difficult, often conflicting choices in medicine, and practitioners are limited in any rebuttal because of confidentiality issues. There is a missed opportunity by the media to comment on the competing allocation of resources across health, to tackle complex issues relating to what we as a society most value in health services, and to canvass whether or not the waiting list for surgical procedures is a sign of a failing system, or a system based on fairness according to priorities of need.

5   Conclusion

This exploration reveals worrying signs of disintegration in the fiduciary relationship between patients and health practitioners. My concern is that we are in danger of threatening the strong, valuable, basic foundations of a healthcare partnership: good medical communication; care and consideration; and respect and dignity. In addition, this demise in trust extends to the delivery of healthcare itself, with a threat to the strong ethos of delivering a public health system based on equity and need within the constraints of available resources.

---

15   Toh, Satchwell and Cohen, "Medical Indemnity," 27.

Bibliography

Bourne, Tom, Joke Vanderhaegen, Renit Vranken, Laure Wynants, Bavo De Cock, Mike Peters, Dirk Timmerman, Ben Van Calster, Maria Jalmbrant, Chantal Van Audenhove. "Doctor's Experiences and Their Perception of the Most Stressful Aspects of Complaints Processes in the UK: an Analysis of Qualitative Survey Data." *BMJ Open* 6:e011711 (2016): n.p. Accessed 20 July 2016, doi:10.1136/bmjopen-2016-011711.

Ganesh, K. "Patient-Doctor Relationship: Changing Perspectives and Medical Litigation." *Indian Journal of Urology* 25.3 (2009): n.p. Accessed 30 July 2016. doi:10.4103/0970-1591.56204.

Hughes, James. "Organization and Information at the Bed-side: The Experience of the Medical Division of Labor University Hospitals' inpatients." PhD diss., University of Chicago, 1995, Chap. One.

Jory, John. "Who's the Boss in the Doctor-Patient Relationship?" *Australian Doctor*, July 7, 2016. Accessed 7 July 2016. http://www.australiandoctor.com.au/smart-practice/in-your-practice/whos-the-boss-in-the-doctor-patient-relationship.

Lateef, Fatimah. "Patient Expectations and the Paradigm Shift of Care in 2016." *Journal of Emergencies, Trauma and Shock*, 4.2 (2011): 163–167. Accessed 27 July, 2016. doi: 10.4103/0974-2700.82199.

Toh, Win-Li, Linda Satchwell, and Jonathan Cohen. "Medical Indemnity – Who's Got the Perfect Cure?" Paper presented to the Institute of Actuaries of Australia at the 12th Accident Compensation Seminar, Melbourne, Victoria, November 22–24, 2004.

CHAPTER 2

Reading the Patient and Reading the Self: an Analysis of the Place of Cultural Theory in Occupational Therapy

Lani R. Stockwell and Scott E. Hendrix

One of the most obvious things to remember about patients is something that is all too often ignored or overlooked—that patients are people embedded in particular cultures, with the messy complexities we all possess. Furthermore, as people, patients pay attention not only to the words healthcare professionals use in dealing with them, but also looks, reactions, and subtle non-verbal cues used in interacting with them. Through these various forms of discourse between practitioner and patient, a reality is being constructed that can either aid in treatment or make treatment more difficult—if not completely impossible. The patient-practitioner relationship is pivotal in both the provision of effective care and patient adherence to a treatment plan.

Many people who enter into healthcare careers do so for altruistic reasons and often express a desire to help others. However, in order to help the patient, one should see that individual as a person, never reduced to 'a body with a set of symptoms.'[1] Patients expect to be treated as partners in the care they receive, but traditional medical education has all too often been one in which practitioners are trained to function as 'body mechanics,' seeing constellations of symptoms rather than people.[2] There have been efforts to combat this attitude, and since the 1960s practitioners have often taken courses in subjects such as medical humanities as part of their training.[3] However, this tends to be true of physicians more often than other health professionals—such as nurses, physical therapists, and occupational therapists—and even when such courses

---

1 Wayne A. Beach, "Patients, Doctors, and Other Helping Relationships," *21st Century Communication: A Reference Handbook*, ed. William F. Eadie, (Los Angeles: Sage Publications, 2009), vol. 1: 358–370, 359–360.

2 Beach, "Patients, Doctors, and Other Helping Relationships," 360; Angela Coulter, "Patients' Expectations," *Medical Education and Training: From Theory to Delivery*, eds. Yvonne Carter and Neil Jackson, (Oxford: Oxford University Press, 2009), 45–58.

3 Howard Brody, "Teaching at the University of Texas Medical Branch, 1971–1974: Humanities, Ethics, or Both?," *The Development of Bioethics in the United States*, eds. Jeremy R. Garrett, Fabrice Jotterand, and D. Christopher Ralston (Dordrecht: Spring, 2013), 25–36.

© KONINKLIJKE BRILL NV, LEIDEN, 2019 | DOI:10.1163/9789004386563_004

are required as part of a medical curriculum, they are often compartmental-
ized, provided as modules within larger courses, or implemented in the early
part of a student's education, which can allow the student to treat the course as
something to be endured and dispensed with rather than a central part of their
education.[4] That is not always the case—as only one example, Carroll University's Master of Occupational Therapy programs requires students to take a
three-course sequence of medical humanities classes; two in their first year of
study and one in their final year. While this educational commitment to medical humanities may be unconventional for a professional program of this sort,
it is in line with a growing trend in medical schools: 69 of 133 accredited medical schools in the U.S. now include at least one such course in their curricula.[5]

These courses take many forms, but one insight of the humanities that can
be of great use for medical professionals is that understanding culture is fundamental to working with patients, and many elements that people think of
as self-evidently "real," such as gender, race, or even whether a condition is
perceived as a medical or social issue, are in fact socially constructed through
a discourse between people that involves both verbal and nonverbal forms of
communication.[6] Michel Foucault (1926-1984) pioneered the field of discourse
theory, and his name is a constant byword in the humanities today, coming up
any time there is a mention of gender, or the study of power relationships or
sexuality, among many other topics.[7] For this current paper, we must narrow
down what Foucault meant by discourse and how one might analyse it. In its
essence, Foucault argued that every word used in communication as well as every instance of nonverbal communication functions as a sign that has meaning
imbued by experiences, attitudes, feelings, and intents of the communicator.[8]
It is important to note that much of the meaning imbued in this sign occurs
through unconscious characteristics of the communicator, but perhaps even

4   Therese Jones, "Oh, the Humanit(ies)!' Dissent, Democracy, and Danger," *Medicine, Health
    and the Arts: Approaches to the Medical Humanities*, eds. Victoria Bates, Alan Bleakley, and
    Sam Goodman (New York: Routledge, 2014), 27–38.
5   Adrianna Banaszek, "Medical Humanities Courses Becoming Prerequisites in Many Med-
    ical Schools," *CMAJ*, 2011 183.8: E441–E442, http://www.ncbi.nlm.nih.gov/pmc/articles/
    PMC3091916/, accessed 20 July 2016.
6   For an excellent discussion of social constructivism as it relates to science, including sci-
    entific medicine, see André Kukla, *Social Constructivism and the Philosophy of Science*
    (New York: Routledge, 2000).
7   For a concise entrée into Foucault's thought, one should start with Paul Rabinow, ed. *The
    Foucault Reader* (New York: Pantheon Books, 1984).
8   For a precis of this approach, see Marianne W Jørgensen and Louise J Phillips, *Discourse Anal-
    ysis as Theory and Method* (London: Sage Publications, 2002), chapters 2 and 3. The rest of
    this paragraph is drawn from this source.

more important is what that sign comes to signify to others. Discourse is a two-way street, and the person to whom communication is directed interprets signs through the lens of his or her own experiences, emotions, educational background, attitudes, and a nearly endless host of other characteristics that affect the signifier as it is received. Thus, a communicator has only partial control over the 'sign' that he or she transmits, and the 'signifier' ultimately received may well be quite different than what the communicator had consciously intended. To further complicate the issue, signs consist of manner of dress, facial expressions, or even a person's gender and how he or she expresses it, at least as often as they consist of spoken words, all filtered through the various lenses of the viewer or listener.[9] According to such theories, culture is built up of these discursive building blocks, and the nonverbal and often unconscious elements are contingent largely upon an individual's culture.

A bare description of these elements of discourse theory may sound unnecessarily complicated or bewildering, and it certainly does point to a reality that is more complicated and messy than many like to consider. It is certainly more complicated than many of the students in Carroll University's Occupational Therapy program think it is when they first start the program, which is why most incoming students consider themselves 'very' or even 'fully' culturally competent, but by the end of their first year of study only 38% would still call themselves 'very' or 'fully' culturally competent. Over 62% of students finishing their first year of study would classify themselves as only 'somewhat' culturally competent.[10] Such results are in line with what was expected when the data were gathered, and is consistent with a growing understanding on the part of the student of the complexities of understanding culture and how it is constituted.[11] However, rather than being discouraged by these complexities, student understanding of the value of cultural competency in healthcare grows markedly during their first year of study when exposed to medical humanities courses. By the end of their first year of study, 59% of Carroll University's Master of Occupational Therapy students report that understanding

---

9   The literature on signs versus signifiers is truly vast and is heavily influenced by the theories of the French psychoanalyst, Jacques Lacan (1901–1981). In addition to Jørgensen and Phillips' study, see Ed Pluth's *Signifiers and Acts: Freedom in Lacan's Theory of the Subject* (Albany: State University of New York Press, 2007), 25–29.

10 Survey results were gathered in June and August of 2016 (see Appendix A).

11 Many researchers have noted this effect of the study of culture on student perceptions. See Klaus Roth, "European Ethnology and Intercultural Communication," *Ethnologia Europaea* 26.1 (1996): 3–16; Angela McRobbie, *The Uses of Cultural Studies: A Textbook* (Thousand Oaks: Sage Publications, 2005), introduction.

cultural characteristics is 'essential' to providing proper care, while another 38% report that it is 'very important.'[12]

In order to understand why students come to see cultural understanding as so important, we will now turn to a concrete example of how discourse analysis and an understanding of culture can function in a real world setting to allow for a better understanding of the relationship between a healthcare professional and her client. In this instance, an Occupational Therapist with seventeen years of health care experience assumed the care of a 43-year-old man with morbid obesity who had been admitted to the emergency department via E.M.S. for a chief complaint of fever, malaise, and lower extremity (LE) pain, oozing, and oedema.[13] It is important to note that the OT was the fourth rehabilitation therapist assigned to this patient, whom we will call 'Ben' for the remainder of the paper. The three previous therapists deferred seeing Ben for reasons documented as being related to his medical status. However, upon medical chart review the OT could find no indication to defer evaluation from a medical standpoint, both on the day she received the order, nor in previous days when the other therapists had deferred Ben.

Whenever it comes to a discursive relationship between individuals, it is essential to understand something about the cultural elements within which they exist. In this instance, both Ben and the therapists assigned to him shared many cultural elements, which definitely had an impact on his care. Of particular importance in this case is how Americans tend to view obesity. 83% of Americans state that those who are obese are 'very' or 'somewhat' responsible for being so, with similar percentages blaming lack of exercise and watching too much television as primary factors.[14] Most of those who are obese report that stigmatization is a common occurrence and even health professionals are susceptible to biases against the obese.[15] In one study, 1/3rd of physicians listed obesity as one of the top diagnostic or social categories likely to make them respond negatively to a patient, while in another study, 63% of nurses attributed obesity to a lack of self-control, while 31% stated that they preferred not to care for obese patients and 28% reported that they were 'repulsed' by obese

---

12   See Appendix A.

13   The Occupational Therapist responsible for the patient in this case study was Dr. Lani Stockwell, who provided the details for use here. For the complete case study, see Appendix B.

14   Robert J. Blendon, Mollyann Brodie, John Benson, and Drew E. Altman, *American Public Opinion and Health Care* (Washington, D.C.: C.Q. Press, 2011), 348–349.

15   J. Myers and J.C. Rosen, "Obesity Stigmatization and Coping: Relation to Mental Health Symptoms, Body image, and Self-esteem," *International Journal of Obesity and Related Metabolic Disorders* 23.3 (1999): 221–230.

persons. 12% of nurses stated that they did not want to touch obese patients at all.[16]

The point about the above statistics is not that a large portion of American medical professionals are heartless when dealing with obese patients. Rather, we should note that the view of these professionals is reflective of the larger society, one that views obesity as a moral issue tied directly to sin.[17] This attitude did not come about overnight. Puritans had an outsized influence on the early development of American culture, and Puritan morality is rooted in the ability to control bodily desires, like hunger. For Puritans, 'universal human depravity' resulted from humankind's fall from grace, and only by adhering to God's law are we able to constrain our depraved natural inclinations toward bodily pleasures, such as gluttony.[18] During the nineteenth century many equated dieting with moral self-control in the face of abundance and the new consumer culture, and during the two World Wars Americans were regularly assailed with moralistic and frequently religious messages calling on people to control their diets.[19] The result is that in modern America, it is common for people (including medical professionals) to see obesity not as a medical condition, but as a moral failing—a view often held by those who are themselves obese.[20]

It would be easy to dismiss such views of obesity if they were not so commonly held in America, and it must be remembered that for most people these ideas are not present as part of their conscious evaluation of the world around them. Rather, these ideas are part of the underlying view of the world that many people hold, representing a filter through which their communications with others pass, and through which all signifiers are received. Reinforced through various forms of discourse—the obese man or woman is typically seen as either asexual or sexualized in some perverse way in Hollywood imagery, and movies that feature 'overweight characters frequently place them in the role of 'jokesters' or 'losers'[21]—negative views of obese people and obesity

16   Rebecca Puhl and Kelly D. Brownell, "Bias, Discrimination, and Obesity," *Obesity Research* 6.12 (2012): 788–805.

17   John Portmann, *A History of Sin: Its Evolution to Today and Beyond* (New York: Rowman and Littlefield, 2007), 128.

18   Louis Groarke, *The Good Rebel: Understanding Freedom and Morality* (Madison: Fairleigh Dickinson University Press, 2002), 135–136.

19   Portmann, *A History of Sin: Its Evolution to Today and Beyond*, 128–130.

20   Roland Littlewood, *Pathologies of the West: An Anthropology of Mental Illness in Europe and America* (Ithaca: Cornell University Press, 2002), 84–86.

21   Frances O'Connor, *Obesity and the Media* (New York: The Rosen Publishing Group, 2009), 38–39; Kathleen LeBesco, *Revolting Bodies?: The Struggle to Redefine Fat Identity* (Amherst: University of Massachusetts Press, 2004), 89–108. There are far too many forms of discourse about obesity in America to be properly analyzed here, from representations

have attained hegemonic status. These views and attitudes are seen as not only normal but also normative, and go both unquestioned and often unrecognized, which can have devastating consequences in healthcare settings.

Turning our attention back to our case study involving Ben's treatment, we can see the impacts of the negative views many people have toward the obese. When the OT assigned to work with Ben contacted his nurse to announce that she planned on visiting him, the nurse replied, 'Are you sure you want to work with him? He stinks. I wouldn't [work with him] if I had the luxury.'[22] She described Ben as 'needy [and] gross,' and suggested the OT get in and out as quickly as possible. These attitudes were not confined to his nurse, as negative comments about Ben were present throughout his chart. More than one healthcare professional indicated that his condition was self-imposed, he was labelled 'unfortunate' too many times to mention, and the word 'lazy' recurred throughout his chart. There were 32 notes of deferral for treatment based on various rationales, more than the occupational therapist had ever observed in her years of professional practice.

Although it is unlikely that any of Ben's healthcare workers used terms such as 'lazy' or 'unfortunate' when speaking to him, there are many avenues of discourse beyond the use of words. Even when a nurse or a therapist uses only the most professional language, tone of voice, reluctance to touch the patient, facial expression, or even haste to finish the assigned task and leave the patient's presence can all function as eloquent signifiers for the patient.[23] Ben clearly understood the messages being relayed to him—during his four weeks of hospitalization, he refused to work with therapists other than the OT assigned to him, and also refused to work with all but four nurses. Perception of self and identity is significantly shaped by societal influence, and indeed in this case, Ben's attitude and perceived non-compliance was largely the result of disaffirmation. The patient's narrative, or experience of illness, was overshadowed by

---

in popular magazines, music, reality television, and even pornography. David W. Haslam, "Obesity and Sexuality," *Controversies in Obesity*, eds. David W. Haslam, Arya M. Sharma, and Carel W. le Roux (London: Springer, 2014), 45–52; Trajce Cvetkovski, *The Pop Music Idol and the Spirit of Charisma: Reality Television Talent Shows in the Digital Economy of Hope* (New York: Palgrave Macmillan, 2015), 24–26.

22   The rest of the information in this paragraph is from the treating OT's case study, which is contained in Appendix A.

23   Robin Tolmach Lakoff, "Nine Ways of Looking at Apologies: The Necessity for Interdisciplinary Theory and Method in Discourse Analysis," *The Handbook of Discourse Analysis*, eds. Deborah Schiffrin, Deborah Tannen, and Heidi E. Hamilton (Malden: Blackwell Publishing, 2001), 199–215.

the dominant narrative of the healthcare culture and medical model viewing disability as a deviation from a reference considered 'normal.'

The importance of understanding the multiple avenues of discourse and how our society constructs hegemonic attitudes about those such as the obese make interdisciplinary courses in medical humanities a vital part of medical education. Not just because it is possible to teach students how discourse functions, but because by pulling the veil back and making this essential element of cultural construction clear, we can hope for better attitudes toward their patients on the part of medical professionals, which in turn lead to better therapeutic outcomes. Howard M. Spiro, the former chief of gastroenterology in the Department of Internal Medicine at Yale, has argued that empathy 'underlies the qualities of the humanistic physician and should frame the skills of all professionals who care for patients.'[24] He pointed to the practice of taking a patient's history as crucial to teaching empathy, for this is where a physician in training can get to know a patient as a person and understand his or her 'story.'[25] There is evidence that empathy can be learned, and such evidence repeatedly highlights the importance of understanding not only why another person might be as he or she is, but also why the individual seeking to learn empathy feels as he or she does.[26]

Students frequently respond well to discussions about cultural construction and how hegemonic notions are built through discourse, even if they are sometimes bewildered at first. As one second year OT student noted: 'Cultural understanding is incredibly important to patient care. A person's culture has a strong influence on their identity, which consists of who they are, what they do and become, and what they believe. If the practitioner does not have some understanding of their patient's culture, how can they properly treat them?'[27] That was certainly true of Ben, from our case study. A breakthrough moment occurred when the OT simply asked about his hobbies and what he liked to do for enjoyment. Ben later admitted that the OT had been the first health care 'person' to ask him what his hobbies were, what he liked to do, and why he did not do them anymore.[28] He said that at first, he wanted to respond that it was

---

24   Howard M. Spiro, "What is Empathy and Can it be Taught?" *Empathy and the Practice of Medicine: Beyond Pills and the Scalpel*, eds. Howard M. Spiro, Mary G. McCrea Curnen, Enid Peschel, and Deborah St. James (New Haven: Yale University Press, 1993), 7–14.

25   Spiro, "What is Empathy and Can it be Taught?," 12–13.

26   Jane Stein-Parbury, *Patient and Person: Interpersonal Skills in Nursing* (New York: Elsevier, 2014, 5th edition), 144–151; Simon Baron-Cohen, *The Science of Evil: On Empathy and the Origins of Cruelty* (New York: Basic Books, 2011), 15–42.

27   See Appendix B.

28   See Appendix A. The rest of the information in this paragraph comes from this source.

not the OT's business, but he decided that he wanted 'someone to know that I wasn't just fat.' Ben ended up following through with the complete plan of care that he and the OT created together on that first day because, in his words, 'it included more than just reprimands.' Ben clearly felt the stigma associated with being obese in American culture. He apologized more than once for being 'in the hospital like this' and for the fact that the OT had to 'be the one to care for him.' It was by recognizing his humanness rather than interacting with the socially constructed category of the obese person that the OT was able to provide successful treatment.

Every patient functions within multiple categories of person. One might be a middle-class white person who grew up in a religious background, which happens to be true of both authors of this paper, a woman working in a professional setting, a man who came from a working-poor background—each of these descriptions is true of one of the authors of this paper—or some combination of these categories, or many more. As Kimberly Crenshaw has argued, none of us are simply one category or another, but a blending of many different categories, and it is this intersectionality that makes people both so interesting as well as so difficult to fully understand.[29]

Bibliography

Banaszek, Adrianna. "Medical Humanities Courses Becoming Prerequisites in Many Medical Schools." *CMAJ,* 2011 183.8: E441–E442, http://www.ncbi.nlm.nih.gov/pmc/articles/PMC3091916/, accessed 20 July 2016.

Baron-Cohen, Simon. *The Science of Evil: On Empathy and the Origins of Cruelty.* New York: Basic Books, 2011.

Beach, Wayne A. "Patients, Doctors, and Other Helping Relationships." *21st Century Communication: A Reference Handbook,* edited by William F. Eadie, volume 1. Los Angeles: Sage Publications, 2009.

Blendon, Robert J., Brodie, Mollyann, Benson, John, and Altman, Drew E. *American Public Opinion and Health Care.* Washington, D.C.: C.Q. Press, 2011.

Brody, Howard. "Teaching at the University of Texas Medical Branch, 1971-1974: Humanities, Ethics, or Both?." In *The Development of Bioethics in the United States,* edited by Jeremy R. Garrett, Fabrice Jotterand, and D. Christopher Ralston. Dordrecht: Spring, 2013.

---

29   Kimberly Crenshaw, "Mapping the Margins: Intersectionality, Identity Politics, and Violence Against Women of Color," *Stanford Law Review* 43.6 (1991): 1241–1299.

Coulter, Angela. "Patients' Expectations." In *Medical Education and Training: From Theory to Delivery*, edited by Yvonne Carter and Neil Jackson. Oxford: Oxford University Press, 2009.

Crenshaw, Kimberlé. "Mapping the Margins: Intersectionality, Identity Politics, and Violence Against Women of Color." *Stanford Law Review*. 43.6 (1991): 1241–1299.

Cvetkovski, Trajce. *The Pop Music Idol and the Spirit of Charisma: Reality Television Talent Shows in the Digital Economy of Hope*. New York: Palgrave Macmillan, 2015.

Groarke, Louis. *The Good Rebel: Understanding Freedom and Morality*. Madison: Fairleigh Dickinson University Press, 2002.

Haslam, David W. "Obesity and Sexuality." *Controversies in Obesity*, edited by David W. Haslam, Arya M. Sharma, and Carel W. le Roux. London: Springer, 2014.

Jones, Therese. "Oh, the Humanit(ies)!' Dissent, Democracy, and Danger." *Medicine, Health and the Arts: Approaches to the Medical Humanities*, edited by Victoria Bates, Alan Bleakley, and Sam Goodman. New York: Routledge, 2014.

Jørgensen, Marianne W and Phillips, Louise J. *Discourse Analysis as Theory and Method*. London: Sage Publications, 2002.

Kukla, André. *Social Constructivism and the Philosophy of Science*. New York: Routledge, 2000.

Lakoff, Robin Tolmach. "Nine Ways of Looking at Apologies: The Necessity for Interdisciplinary Theory and Method in Discourse Analysis." In *The Handbook of Discourse Analysis*, edited by Deborah Schiffrin, Deborah Tannen, and Heidi E. Hamilton. Malden: Blackwell Publishing, 2001.

LeBesco, Kathleen. *Revolting Bodies?: The Struggle to Redefine Fat Identity*. Amherst: University of Massachusetts Press, 2004.

Littlewood, Roland. *Pathologies of the West: An Anthropology of Mental Illness in Europe and America*. Ithaca: Cornell University Press, 2002.

McRobbie, Angela. *The Uses of Cultural Studies: A Textbook*. Thousand Oaks: Sage Publications, 2005.

Myers, J., and Rosen, J.C. "Obesity Stigmatization and Coping: Relation to Mental Health Symptoms, Body image, and Self-esteem." *International Journal of Obesity and Related Metabolic Disorders* 23.3 (1999): 221–230.

O'Connor, Frances. *Obesity and the Media*. New York: The Rosen Publishing Group, 2009.

Portmann, John. *A History of Sin: Its Evolution to Today and Beyond*. New York: Rowman and Littlefield, 2007.

Pluth, Ed. *Signifiers and Acts: Freedom in Lacan's Theory of the Subject*. Albany: State University of New York Press, 2007.

Puhl, Rebecca, and Brownell, Kelly D. "Bias, Discrimination, and Obesity." *Obesity Research* 6.12 (2012): 111–136.

Rabinow, Paul, ed. *The Foucault Reader*. New York: Pantheon Books, 1984.

Roth, Klaus. "European Ethnology and Intercultural Communication." *Ethnologia Europaea* 26.1 (1996): 3–16.

Spiro, Howard M. "What is Empathy and Can it be Taught." *Empathy and the Practice of Medicine: Beyond Pills and the Scalpel*, edited by Howard M. Spiro, Mary G. McCrea Curnen, Enid Peschel, and Deborah St. James. New Haven: Yale University Press, 1993.

Stein-Parbury, Jane. *Patient and Person: Interpersonal Skills in Nursing.* New York: Elsevier, 2014.

Appendix A
Q.1

Age, gender and life-cycle factors must be considered in interactions with individuals and families (e.g., high value placed on the decision of elders, the role of eldest male or female in families, or roles and expectation of children within the family).

· **Answered: 29**

Answer Choices–

Responses–

–

Never true

0.00%

0

–

Occasionally true

0.00%

0

–

Often true

31.03%

9

–

Always true

68.97%

20

Total

29

Considering family members, especially in the practice of OT, is extremely beneficial since families will implement treatment plans.

Different genders, generations, and factors of life may all pose different beliefs from person to person.

Very important to acknowledge factors that the client considers important, shows you have concern for their beliefs. Helps establish a therapeutic relationship.

Cultural factors should always be considered when interacting with individuals and families, especially in health care. Culture greatly influences communication styles, as well as treatment goals.

It is important to consider age, gender, and life-cycle factors, because these things may differ widely between cultures. Practitioners must not assume that all of their patients are the same in this regard.

We often understand our roles in society from our roles in our family.

These will significantly affect how you treat the patient.

It is always important to ask the patient what is important to them.

Age, gender, and life-cycle factors will always play a significant role in dictating overall interactions between clinicians and providers.

Each culture varies and the Hispanic culture is very family based and take care of and greatly respect their elders.

Different cultural viewpoints can vary regarding this statement.

Q. 2

The meaning or value of medical treatment and health education may vary greatly among cultures.

· Answered: 29

Answer Choices–

Responses–

–

Never true

0.00%

0

–

Occasionally true

0.00%

0

–

Sometimes true

6.90%

2

–

Always true

93.10%

27

Total

29

Every culture views healthcare and treatment different. If you do not know enough about a culture, being competent enough to ask is very beneficial.

There are many different cultures who will have different views on proper medical treatment. Within those cultures are subcultures, which may also play a role in their treatment beliefs.

If the client believes there is no meaning to the treatment he/she is being prescribed they will be less likely to continue treatment or follow directions when the healthcare provider is considered uneducated.

Different cultures have differing values and beliefs, which includes their value in medicine and health education. Some cultures may value the roles of their families and community members as the primary caretakers in medical treatment situations.

We have learned that it is critical of healthcare professionals to not only educate their patients, but to ensure they have understood what is being told to them.

The culture of medicine is different around the world.

In many cultures western medicine is not typical and medical treatment is not valued as highly. They may trust doctors more or less and follow through with treatment more or less depending on their culture.

It is important to find out the patient's values and believes when it comes to medical treatment and health education. Even very similar cultures vary in how they value certain aspects of medical treatments and health education.

Some cultures do not seek Western Medicine because they do not believe it will work. Individuals who live in a lower SES area may not understand the medical language used and fear asking questions due to the possibly being seen as nonintelligent.

Q. 3

Religion and health care beliefs may influence how individuals and families respond to illnesses, disease and death.

· **Answered: 29**

Answer Choices–

Responses–

–

Never true

0.00%

0

–

Occasionally true

0.00%

0

–

Sometimes true

24.14%

7

–

Always true

75.86%

22

Total

29

Especially in palliative care and hospice care.

Some religions don't believe in medical treatment at all; they may choose to forego medical treatment even in life threatening situations if they have strong beliefs toward that specific religion.

If the health care treatment prescribed contradicts a client's beliefs, they are much less likely to take part in the treatment.

Some individuals may greatly value religion and leave their fate up to a higher power instead of seeking common medical care for illnesses or disease.

Practitioners must understand that some religions do not believe in medical treatment, such as Jehovah's Witnesses, who do not believe in blood transfusions.

I think religion plays a role in this. Religion helps formulate what happens after life. This can give people different perceptions on illness and death.

For some clients, religion may be at the centre of their care but some clients' religion will have no influence.

Certain religions prohibit treatments such as blood transfusions.

Religion often effects beliefs regarding life after death.

I do not want to say always because it depends on the patient, but even if the patient claims to have no religious beliefs that will still influence their responses to illness, death, and disease.

Q. 4

Cultural understanding is [insert your answer here] to patient care.

Answer Choices–

Responses–

–

Unimportant

0.00%

0

–

Of little importance

0.00%

0

–

Of considerable importance

27.59%

8

Is of central importance

72.41%

21

Total

29

Q. 5

When considering how to provide successful patient care, keeping abreast of the major health concerns and issues for ethnically and racially diverse client populations residing in the geographic locale where I will practice ...

Answer Choices–

Responses–

–

is unimportant

0.00%

0

–

is of some small importance

0.00%

0

–

is very important

31.03%

9

–

is essential

68.97%

20

Total

29

Q. 6

Being well versed in the most current and proven practices, treatments and interventions for major health problems among ethnically and racially diverse groups
within the geographic locale where I will practice ...

Answer Choices–

Responses–

–

is unimportant

0.00%

0

–

is of some small importance

3.45%

1

–

is very important

37.93%

11

–

is essential

58.62%

17

Total

29

Q. 7

How important is cultural understanding to patient care?

· **Answered: 29**

· **Skipped: 0**

Being culturally proficient, or aware of other cultures that may be present, is of
upmost importance in patient care. Understanding how patients will react and continue treatment care greatly impacts healthcare.

  Considerably important

  Cultural understanding is extremely important to patient care. In order to provide holistic services, one must be aware of the patient's background, including his
or her cultural beliefs.

  Essential in establishing a client centred, therapeutic relationship.

  Cultural understanding is essential to patient care. Occupational therapy is
client-centred and occupational based. This means the client and their occupations
is the basis of the therapy process. Without a true consideration of our patient's
cultural background we cannot adhere to the very nature of our profession.

Cultural understanding is crucial to quality patient care. In order to practice client centred care, the health professional must become aware of and seek to understand diverse cultures. Diverse cultures can affect communication styles, assessment strategies, intervention methods, and patient goals.

It is extremely important.

Essential

Cultural understanding is crucial to providing client centred care. As practitioners having knowledge about other cultures helps to improve the practitioner-patient relationship.

Extremely important

is of considerable importance, especially when building rapport with clients.

Cultural understanding is incredibly important to patient care. A person's culture has a strong influence on their identity, which consists of who they are, what they do, and what they believe. If the practitioner does not have some understanding of their patient's culture, how can they properly treat them?

Crucial. Cultural beliefs and values play a key role in determining patient care and how patients will react to health care services.

It is crucial to provide the best care possible.

Very important

Extremely important

It is very important. Perceptions and ideologies differ among cultures. In order to set proper expectations, cultural understanding is necessary.

Extremely important, a health care professional needs to be aware of the patient's culture to provide the best care.

It is vital to understand one's own culture as well as clients' culture because of the many factors that culture impacts; for example, clients who communicate differently may come across as non-compliant to the practitioner when it's really an issue of communication. Understanding a client's culture helps the practitioner better understand the client's values.

It is essential when providing the best care to patients.

Cultural understand/proficiency is at the core of providing best patient care.

Extremely important

Cultural understanding is essential to patient care and provides optimal results for your patient. It increases compliance and rapport between the patient and practitioner.

It is crucial particularly in client-centred practices.

It is as important as the client, highly important.

Without question, understanding a patient's culture is essential to effective, meaningful, and client-centred care.

Extremely important. By understanding culture you are able to provide better care to the patient.

It is vital. The first step in treating a patient is understanding their culture.

It is essential to patient care. Understanding a patient's culture will allow you to be culturally competent. This will help the patient feel more comfortable and satisfied with their care.

Q. 8

What cultural factors should a healthcare practitioner consider? Why those factors?
· **Answered: 29**
· **Skipped: 0**

Any cultural factor that impacts healthcare such as healing, other members of the culture that provide treatment and spiritual beliefs all need to be incorporated. If a practitioner can incorporate other members of a culture this may be beneficial to treatment.

The culture's views on health and well-being is most important for a healthcare practitioner in the heathcare setting. Other settings may be different.

Language, religion, ses, ethnicity, age, gender, education, past life experiences and upbringing. These factors are all essential to understanding who the person is and why they do the things they do. It is pertinent information when trying to create a treatment plan for an individual that they will want to do and will stick to.

What member of the family makes decisions. Religious beliefs (time, food, clothing, treatment). Communication issues (verbal, nonverbal).

A healthcare practitioner should consider cultural factors such as religion, language, tradition, familial roles and so forth. These are not the only cultural factors a healthcare practitioner should consider; however, these factors can aid the healthcare practitioner in building rapport with the patient.

Healthcare practitioners should consider many cultural factors including gender, race, socioeconomic status, age, religion, and possibly marriage status. These factors create uniqueness for a person as well as personal identity. These factors may affect the relationship between the patient and caregiver, and are essential to providing the best care.

age, ethnicity, geography, gender, socioeconomic status, disability

Religion, family life, ethnic practices

Religion, ethnic background, family dynamic, and cultural practices are important to understand in order to be culturally sensitive and provide care that is specific to that patient's values and beliefs.

Understanding subcultures, since it gives insight into preferred occupation.

They should consider family dynamics and role of each family member because many cultures places family values at a very high priority.

A healthcare practitioner should consider a patient's values, beliefs, language, religion, SES, geographical location, gender, sexuality, and, family style, amongst others. All of these factors have a significant impact on the patient's life and can influence their ability to participate in treatment. The healthcare practitioner must look at the patient holistically, considering these factors and the influence that they may have on the patient.

SES, educational status, religion. I believe SES is crucial to understanding patients and how they view health care. Also understanding their educational level will help formulate patient interaction. Also, for question 9, I think one should be able to type in their answer since I wanted to put "not at all" although I have experience with culture because no one can ever be fully culturally competent.

Religion, Socioeconomic status, Education, Geographical location. These factors will help the practitioner to better understand their client and help frame their course of treatment in a client-centred fashion.

Religion, the patient and family's views on health and wellness, sickness and disease, and the role family has in the patient's life. These factors shape an individual's values and beliefs and makes them unique to the culture they may identify with.

Beliefs, other ways of care, spiritual beliefs for after life or present life, and other care techniques. These factors are crucial because they will help the patient better trust the practitioner, when the practitioner has knowledge of culture and some aspects of the culture. Discussing the cultural factors with the patient, shows the patient how much the practitioner cares about the health of the patient.

Language, poverty, religious beliefs

Family roles, religion, beliefs, and gender roles. A health care provider should consider all of these factors because they may be important to the client.

There are numerous factors practitioners to consider, such as race, gender, education level, and healthcare values. Factors such as these help practitioners better understand clients' behaviours, beliefs, comfort level, possible biases, and knowledge about health/well-being. By considering these factors, practitioners can provide better care.

Many cultural factors should be considered. These can include: age, ethnicity, religion, gender/sex, marital status, geographical location, and many others depending on what treatment the practitioner will provide. These factors influence the patient's motivation, knowledge about their health, their possible roles in life, values, and beliefs that could influence their overall healthcare.

All factors need to be considered. Everything from age, gender, sexual orientation, SEC, and religion. clients will also have unique personal cultures which play a huge impact on treatment and need to be considered as well.

Race, socioeconomic status, religious beliefs. They will affect how patients perceive you and how they prefer to receive their care.

They should consider how much they value medicine, what their normal medical treatments would consist of, how they communicate and who should be involved in the treatment. This will allow you to frame your treatment in a way that will be the most successful to that patient.

Religion, geographic location, gender, past experiences. These are of particular importance in the U.S. healthcare due to social structures.

Ethnicity, age, religion, region, socioeconomic status, etc. They are important in understanding the client and helps to determine an individualized treatment plan that is meaningful to the client.

It is important for a clinician to consider a patient's beliefs (both spiritual and otherwise), values, language, and socioeconomic status. These factors, while not an exhaustive list, are perhaps some of the most powerful factors that influence a person's interaction with not only a provider, but with medicine in general.

Age, gender, religion, ethnicity, language. These factors are of the most importance because they give the health care provider a greater understand of the individual. For example, in certain cultures women are not allowed to address men other than their husband, so if a woman is present in the room of this culture, it is important to know that the health care provider cannot address the women till her husband arrives.

Personal, family, and religious beliefs and language are some of the cultural factors a healthcare practitioner should consider. These factors stress what is important to the patient and allows a better understanding of a patient's view towards health care and other beliefs. Language is important when communicating with a patient in order to know what they are able to comprehend, understand, and articulate.

Religion, Race, Ethnicity, Language. They can be a part of the patient's identity. Disregarding the factors that define the patient will lead to poor understanding and care.

Q. 9.

How cultural competent are you?
· **Answered: 29**
· **Skipped: 0**
Answer Choices–
Responses–

–

Not at all.
0.00%
0

–

Somewhat.
62.07%

18

–

Very culturally competent.

34.48%

10

–

I am fully culturally competent.

3.45%

   1

   Total

   29

Appendix B

Case Study #1: Balance between rights of practitioner and patient rights-

The focus of this study is perhaps on the beliefs and values of the practitioner—and the right to recuse from a patient case if the provider has a personal moral conflict with his/her patient. I have witnessed this occurring many times re the care of patients who are obese. I love reading case studies about rights versus responsibilities versus duties— in particular, the ethical principle of beneficence which obviously is protecting others, preventing harm, offering kindness. Beneficence is the first principle of the Occupational Therapy Code of Ethics. In my experience, aversion to the patient's condition has largely been the catalyst for such instances where care is withdrawn and therefore the patient's personhood is overruled by his/her condition and/or medical status.

Case Study: Ben

History of Presenting Illness (HPI): 43 y.o. man with morbid obesity admitted to the ED via EMS for chief complaint of fever, malaise, and lower extremity (LE) pain, oozing and oedema. Per report, patient states that he had not been feeling well for duration approximately two weeks prior to admission. Patient first noticed a weight gain of around 15#, which he states increased to 25# within past two-week period. Rapid weight gain accompanied by fatigue. Bilateral LE oedema resulting in copious drainage which the patient reports as "off colour." Patient febrile upon admission (102.6 degrees) with evident bilateral LE presentation as noted above. Admission weight per digital in-bed scale once on the medical unit was 487 lbs.

Past Medical History (PMH): type 2 diabetes, morbid obesity, chronic venous insufficiency, hypertension, cellulitis, multiple hospital admissions for similar events, lymphedema, anxiety, depression.

Occupational Therapy Evaluation and Assessment
Evaluation:

Prior Level of Function (PLOF)

Activities of Daily Living (ADL)

- *Dressing*: Independent upper body dressing, dependent LB dressing (patient reports he does not don shoes or socks as he is unable to reach lower body. Patient reports that he wears an oversized robe as primary clothing.
- *Bathing*: performed standing at kitchen sink, independent with UB, uses kitchen tongs to clean peri area, cleans lower extremities "by pouring water over legs" while standing on a towel.
- *Grooming*: independent seated at kitchen table with portable basin as needed.
- *Eating*: independent with self-feeding, cooking ("microwave meals, delivery pizza, and mostly sandwiches").
- *Community Access*: patient does not drive as he "cannot fit into car." Uses online service for grocery delivery.
- *Occupations*: reading, computers, "used to love working with electronics."

Of note, patient expressing desire to "go back to school to get (his) MBA" when able but reports "embarrassment and feeling nervous" about going out in a public setting.

Mobility

- Patient owns a rolling walker but does not use. Patient states that he has "no room to use (his) walker" and holds onto "furniture" to help him walk when he feels "unsteady."

Home Layout

- Third floor apartment with elevator access
- Apartment accessible and without stairs to enter
- Bathroom setup: tub/shower which patient does not use. Patient reports that his bathtub is "filled with books" because he doesn't have "any storage space."
- Standard toilet with raised toilet seat attachment; no grab bars

Of note, patient self-identifies as being a hoarder and describes his home environment as being a "series of trails from room to room."

Social History

- Lives alone
- Estranged from family per patient
- Patient does not "get out of the house" and is self-reported as "homebound"
- Unable to identify social supports

Present level of function: Patient requires maximum assistance (x3 persons) for supine to sit EOB. Patient unable to stand secondary to increased pain in bilateral LE's once in dependent position seated EOB.

Of note: patient's lower extremities began to rapidly ooze bloody fluid once seated EOB. RN notified and patient returned to supine with bilateral LE's elevated.

Assessment

Patient presents with impoverished daily routines likely related to constraints of his home living environment, decreased ROM and strength with relationship to increased body habitus, decreased activity tolerance, and physical inability to provide appropriate self-care. Patient unable to physically access community which is a concern as this is a likely contributor to his psychosocial status, anxiety, and further inclination to remain homebound. Patient will benefit from occupational therapy services to facilitate improved capacity for self-care and education toward compensatory strategies to ease self-care task performance and improve functional mobility, promote safety, and target energy conservation. Education will focus on self-management strategies including attention to hygiene and management of clinical conditions, strength and ROM home exercise plan, and restructuring of routines to promote engagement in meaningful life activities and access to community.

Background Information

Excess fat and skin interferes with lymphatic drainage which compromises the immune system. Patients then have recurrent cellulitis and are at great risk for infection. Skin gets sclerotic and thick which contributes to poor circulation (poor oxygenation) and thus the patient is susceptible to pressure ulcers but has an inability to heal wounds. It's an unfortunate viscous cycle.

In patients who present like Ben, the lymph system actually becomes overloaded and cannot hold the fluid so it is literally expelled and flows out of the pores in the skin. In his case, the fluid had a foul odor which caused his hospital room to smell and obviously contribute to the bias and context of this case.

Context of Case—Health Care Environment

I was the fourth rehabilitation therapist to receive Ben on my caseload. The three previous therapists deferred seeing Ben for reasons documented as being related to his medical status. I could not find any reasons to defer OT evaluation from a medical standpoint both on the day I received the order, nor in previous days when he was deferred by my colleagues.

Upon contacting Ben's nurse to let her know that I planned to see her patient, she replied, "Are you sure you want to work with him? He stinks. I wouldn't if I had the luxury." She further went on to state that she was the only nurse on shift who was "crazy enough to treat him." She described Ben as "needy, gross, and "takes too much time" and said, "try to get in and get out."

I found Ben to be none of those. While is room did smell, it was expected and certainly unavoidable. He was initially apologetic about his condition and going so far as to express embarrassment that he was "in the hospital like this" and that I had to "be the one to care for him." He was clearly deconditioned and I would call him broken and defeated. Over the course of 4 weeks, he went from being unable to tolerate sitting on the edge of bed, to standing, walking, and at the end of the month, was able to take a seated shower—in the actual shower—with my help. With the use of long-handled adaptive equipment that I gave him and taught him how to use, he was able to don underwear for the first time in 5 years! (albeit hospital underwear special ordered but nevertheless!). In the end, he demonstrated self-pacing strategies so that he could compensate for his intolerance of activity but all the while still be able to perform simple grooming and hygiene tasks, shower, and take a short walk on the unit using a walker (again I had special ordered for him due to his size). I worked extensively with the case manager to find and set up resources so that his care could continue once discharged. A social worker was also identified for home-based treatment toward finding resources to help Ben access the community and utilize resources to help him participate in the things he wanted to do.

This case is significant because it really emphasizes the power health care practitioners have over their patients. That Ben's first inclination was to apologize for his condition was evidence of that. The therapeutic relationship that developed during our OT sessions was simply due to mutual respect and interest in the humanness of each of us. Unfortunately, Ben refused to work with all other therapists and all but four nurses during the 4-week admission but I can't say as I blame him seeing how he was treated. I was also surprised at the negativity I saw throughout the written documents in Ben's chart. That Ben's condition was self-imposed. He was labelled "unfortunate" too many times to mention. I did see reference to "lazy" as well.

Ben later shared that I had been the first health care "person" to ask him what his hobbies were, what he liked to do, and why he didn't do them anymore. He said that at first, he wanted to tell me that it wasn't my business, but he decided that he wanted "someone to know that I wasn't just fat." Ben ended up following through with all the plan of care that we created together on that first day because "it included more than just reprimands" per Ben.

Once Ben was discharged, I reviewed his chart one last time. I counted 32 notes of deferral for treatment based on various excuses (some were likely legitimate, at least I hope). I have never seen that many in all of my career in a patient whose medical status was relatively stable throughout admission.

However, if we truly wish to understand people—and every patient is a person, not just a constellation of symptoms—it is important to make the effort to understand. Doing so requires borrowings from the humanities, such as the insights of discourse analysis and social constructivism, which can only be fully implemented when combined with the knowledge that healthcare professionals bring to the table. However, when these different disciplines share their knowledge with one another, the result can be both more humane treatment of patients as well as more positive treatment outcomes.

CHAPTER 3

Mandalas of Emotions as Add-on Therapy for Self-Healing and Resolution of Internal Conflicts in Cancer Treatment

Gabriela Salim Spagnol, Li Hui Ling and Li Li Min

1 Cancer Triggers Emotional Conflicts

Cancer remains one of the leading causes of death worldwide.[1] In 2005, approximately 7 million lives were lost to cancer globally, ranking as the second cause of death in many countries, after cardiovascular diseases.[2] According to Ma and Yu (2006),[3] older people are most susceptible to cancer. Along with the population aging, incidence rates will continuously increase in the future, especially in developing countries, with an estimative of up to 15 million new cases in 2020.[4] In low- and middle-income countries, the foreseeable increase in the cancer burden will be even more profound.[5] As developing countries succeed in achieving lifestyles similar to those in advanced economies, they will also face much higher cancer rates, particularly cancers of the breast, colon, prostate and uterus (endometrial carcinoma).[6]

Cancer and its treatment trigger emotional conflicts, which may negatively impact on treatment evolution. During the last decades, the mention of this disease was shrouded by an atmosphere of fear and uncertainty, due to the high rates of death and lack of effective treatments. Even though survival rates have increased, challenges imposed by the treatment, such as hair loss, immunosuppression, associated diseases and physical frailty, bring a great psychological burden to the patient and family. For this reason, add-on therapies

---

1 Panos Kanavos, "The Rising Burden of Cancer in the Developing World," *Annals of Oncology* 17 (2006): 23.

2 Ibid.

3 Xiaomei Ma and Herbert Yu Ma, "Global Burden of Cancer," *Yale Journal of Biology and Medicine* 79 (2006): 86.

4 Panos Kanavos, "The Rising Burden of Cancer in the Developing World," 25.

5 Frank A. Sloan and Hellen Gelband, *Cancer Control Opportunities in Low- and Middle-Income Countries* (Washington, DC: National Academies Press, 2007), 20–65.

6 Ibid.

© KONINKLIJKE BRILL NV, LEIDEN, 2019 | DOI:10.1163/9789004386563_005

play an important role in improving the ability to cope as well as levels of self-esteem, which are issues that are limited and often neglected.

In this sense, the technique "Dialogue with emotions through mandalas" has been applied in order to promote higher awareness of emotions and coping with the disease. Dr. Ling developed the method called "Dialogue with emotions" with a reference to Traditional Chinese Medicine (TCM), aiming to improve recognition and understanding of emotions, and raising self-awareness in order to deal with internal conflicts.[7]

2   Ecological Harmony through the Eyes of Traditional Chinese Medicine

For over 5000 years, members of the Chinese ancient civilization believed that the human being is equal to a miniature universe that functions the same way as nature with its seasonality. For this reason, human beings are considered microcosms in which movements occur just like the changing of the five seasons: spring, summer, high summer, autumn and winter.

The Traditional Chinese Medicine bases its concepts on these five movements, as well as in the functional rhythm of the body, that symbolizes the integration of cycle of plants with changes of seasons, and which are represented by colours and related to different functional systems of the human body. For instance, upon the arrival of spring, plants sprout green; by summer time, the red colour refers to the heat and higher temperatures; and the height of summer when the earth provides the harvest, is represented by yellow, in a reference to fertility. Fall, in turn, is depicted in white, as the temperature drops, and, finally, winter as black, due to lack of sun light. In relation to the human body, green is related to the functional system of the liver, red to the heart, yellow to spleen and pancreas, white to lungs and black to the kidneys.

The definition of well-being of the TCM comprises not only the absence of physical complaints, but a complete harmony in regard to the physical, emotional and mental spheres. Variations of feelings and emotions are part of the human universe. According to the TCM, emotions express the relation with the body and the mind and provide a bridge to access the abilities of self-healing.[8]

---

7   Li Hui Ling, *Dialogando com as Emoções e Promovendo a Saúde* (Curitiba: Insight, 2013), 5–40.
8   Ibid.

The use of stones with a reference to traditional Chinese medicine is a symbolic way to access the emotional level of the human being, and at the same time to cognitively train the abilities related to intuition, creativity and imagination. TCM applies the idea of movement, the art of navigating in a world where every aspect presents two opposite poles, positive and negative, male and female, yin and yang.

3   Translating the Ancient Knowledge

The Mandalas of Emotions applies the Chinese concept of the five movements, five emotions, five colours (green – liver, red – heart, yellow – spleen, white – lungs, black – kidney), Ying/Yang and five directions, providing a composition of stones according to the patient needs. This technique uses five coloured stones the size of a walnut, each of which represents a connection with the universe, according to the five seasons defined by TCM. A relation to the five functional systems (liver, heart, spleen and pancreas, lungs and kidney) is established. These systems work as a network and changing one of the five variables alters the other. Therefore, the Mandalas of Emotions establishes the relation between these five aspects and the emotions, as well as its opposites, as depicted in Figure 3.1.

Depending on the patient needs, one of the five emotions is chosen and stones are placed in a composition, as depicted in Figure 3.2.

The stones are placed around the patient or on his/her abdomen, depending on the self-perceived personality type, according to the classification: 1) intuitive – location: feet; 2) emotive – location: abdomen; 3) rational – location: head.

While relaxing with these stones, patients are guided to connect with their interior, awakening the possibility of self-healing and resilience (see Figure 3.3). According to Ling, this healing corresponds to a new awareness, a new attitude towards life situations. During this treatment, patients report sensations that may include: tingling, heat, pulsation or awakening of certain memories.[9]

The method does not intend to make a diagnosis and treatment of disease (see overleaf a summary of instructions of how to apply mandalas). It is important to remember that in traditional Chinese medicine well-being is a state of harmony between emotion and physical body. By restructuring the emotional aspect, the body will also respond.

---

9   Ibid.

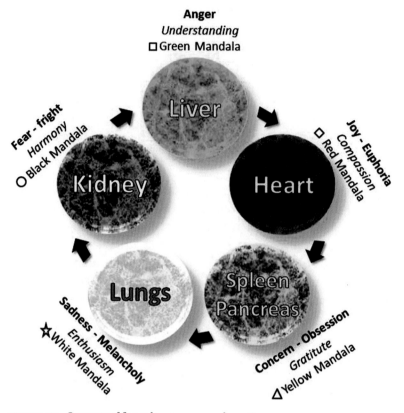

FIGURE 3.1 Concepts of five colours, organs and emotions.

How to apply Mandalas of Emotions?

1) Take a deep dive in the five emotions:
- *anger/understanding,*
- *joy & euphoria/compassion,*
- *concern & obsession/gratitude,*
- *sadness & melancholy/enthusiasm,*
- *fear & fright/harmony.*
- *Welcome the first emotion that comes in your mind, do not try to justi-fy or rationalize.*
- *Do not deny it, nor reject, just feel and welcome. See emotions as a way of learning.*[10]

---

10   Brief instructions to apply Mandalas of Emotions. © 2016 Mandalas of Emotions. Used with permission.

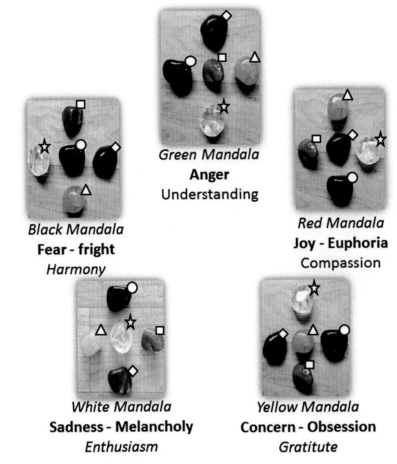

Green Mandala
Anger
Understanding

Black Mandala
Fear - fright
Harmony

Red Mandala
Joy - Euphoria
Compassion

White Mandala
Sadness - Melancholy
Enthusiasm

Yellow Mandala
Concern - Obsession
Gratitute

FIGURE 3.2 Different composition of stones for each emotion.

4   Single Case Study

The patient was a 44-year-old Brazilian woman diagnosed with neuroendo-crine tumour in the left breast in 2004. Neuroendocrine tumours (NET s) are neoplasms that arise from cells of the endocrine (hormonal) and nervous sys-tems.[11] Several issues help define appropriate treatment of a neuroendocrine tu-mour, including its location, invasiveness, hormone secretion, and metastasis.

---

11   Keith Langley, "The Neuroendocrine Concept Today," *Annals of the New York Academy of Sciences* 733 (1994): 1–17.

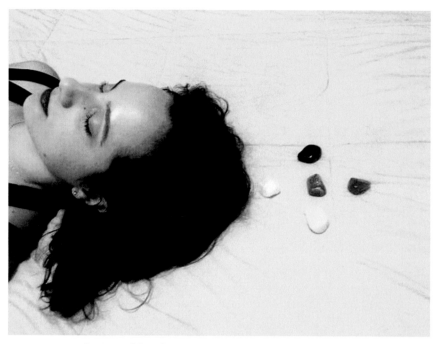

FIGURE 3.3 Applying mandalas of emotions (green mandala).

Treatments may be aimed at curing the disease or at relieving symptoms (palliative care). Clinical follow-up may be feasible for non-functioning low grade neuroendocrine tumours, whereas intermediate and high-grade tumours (non carcinoids) are usually best treated by various early interventions (active therapy) rather than clinical follow-up. Treatments and outcomes have improved over the last decades. In malignant carcinoid tumours, the median survival rate has improved from two years to more than eight years.[12]

With regard to the patient in this report, she was prescribed an immediate mastectomy followed by radiotherapy in 2004, which proved to be effective at that time. However, in April 2013, a cancer recurrence was detected as a metastasis in the right adrenal and kidney, and small foci in lung and mediastinum. The patient was treated with injections of sandostatin during 18 months, a period in which clinical conditions remained stable. Also, the patient received two cycles of treatment with lutetium. After the second cycle, the patient had

---

12   Kjell Öberg and Daniel Castellano, "Current Knowledge on Diagnosis and Staging of Neuroendocrine Tumors," *Cancer and Metastasis Reviews* 30 (2011): 3–7.

a relapse. Two cancer foci were detected, one with a slow growth and another more aggressive in the mediastinum.

During the first semester of 2014, the patient started a treatment with Dr. Li Hui Ling, using Traditional Chinese Medicine. For a year, Dr. Ling provided this treatment once a week or once every two weeks by applying acupuncture. This treatment assisted the patient to re-establish a physical, mental and emotional balance as well as an increase in disposition. In October 2014, the patient started chemotherapy with cisplatin and etoposide, which proved efficient against the most aggressive tumour. During the first half of 2015, Dr. Ling began to apply the mandalas of emotions. This technique allowed the patient to build self-awareness in regard to her emotions, body and mind. Accordingly, there were rapid improvements in physical and emotional crises. In this sense, physical breakdowns related to emotional issues decreased as the patient's emotional resilience increased.

Ten months later, in August 2015, the patient had a relapse, with a stenosis at the entrance of the right lung. The suggested treatment with cisplatin chemotherapy and etoposide was ineffective. In December 2015, the physician prescribed preventive chemotherapy with xeloda and intermodal. Platelet and leukocyte levels decreased significantly and clinical conditions were stabilised.

Yet, in the last week of December (2015), *petechiae* (pinpoint flat round red spots under the skin surface caused by intradermal haemorrhage) were detected in the legs and feet, and platelets fell to 6,000 units per microliter of circulating blood (normally, you have anywhere from 150,000 to 450,000). The patient then stayed at the hospital on three occasions to receive four platelet transfusions. After the last hospitalization, the patient suffered panic attacks. The first episode began with extreme fear, shortness of breath and rapid heartbeat and lasted about 10 min. The patient was afraid of dark and enclosed places, but her physician felt that medication for panic attack was not an option due to the patient's clinical conditions. At that time, she self-discharged from the hospital because of panic attacks.

At home, Dr. Ling applied ME to countermeasure the feeling of fear. With a set of techniques, such as acupuncture, floral therapy and especially the stones placed as mandalas (with a frequent use of black and white mandalas), it was possible to re-establish a state of balance, during a process of self-awareness, sustaining the understanding of the healing process, which provided a clinical improvement and the reestablishment of platelet production by the bone marrow. The full confidence in Dr. Ling and her method is closely related to the patient's resilience, her constant emotional growth, and self-knowledge.

The patient was also instructed to use the mandalas of emotions at home, in order to sustain her welfare, avoiding thus the need to stay at the hospital.

Physical breakdowns related to emotional issues decreased as the patient's emotional resilience increased.

One week after the panic attack, platelets returned and rose slowly but steadily. In regard to the treatment with mandalas, the patient had presented unresolved matters related to emotional issues, which appeared as panic attacks. For this reason, the last and intensive intervention with mandalas after the panic attack focused on the understanding of emotions to improve coping mechanisms, as the patient states in the following transcript:

> I am glad to be at home and without medication. I am sure that my recovery will be more effective and fast. Mandalas are used daily with the help of Dr. Ling, considering my perception of emotions or physical frailty. They became an automatic tool embodied in my routine, and they help me to achieve balance and health.

5   Discussion

During cancer treatment, quality of life and self-esteem may decline considerably due to its great psychological burden. In this sense, strategies like add-on therapies are essential to avoid psychological breakdown that may compromise clinical improvement. Many side effects remain not only during active cancer treatment, but also for a short period thereafter, which can impact on psychological issues. The majority of disease-free cancer survivors report good quality of life one year post treatment, but still a significant number of survivors describe lower overall physical well-being than those who had never experienced cancer.[13]

Medical institutions have continuously worked on establishing standards for quality, patient-centred cancer care that include recommendations for palliative care, distress management, and survivorship care planning.[14] These guidelines focus on comprehensive survivorship care, including support for health behaviour changes, and the assessment and management of the long-term and late effects of cancer and its treatment. Despite improvements in cancer treatment and survivor rates, many challenges remain. Miller and colleagues (2016) state that "future research should also focus on identifying the best methods

13   Kimberly D. Miller, Rebecca L. Siegel and Ahmedin Jemal, "Cancer Statistics 2016," *CA: A Cancer Journal for Clinicians* 66 (2016): 271–289.
14   Sloan and Gelband, *Cancer Control Opportunities in Low- and Middle-Income Countries*, 25.

for encouraging cancer survivors to adopt and maintain a healthy lifestyle".[15] In terms of emotions, many survivors suffer from a fear of recurrence.

In our case study, the patient faced a recurrence nearly ten years after her primary cancer. At this point, unresolved emotional issues came to the surface as panic attacks, compromising the treatment adherence and effectiveness. From our perspective, the major role of mandalas of emotions in this case was to promote greater self-awareness, through an understanding of emotional conflicts. The patient was able to cognitively approach these barriers during self-reflection mediated by stones placed as mandalas symbolizing each emotion she was experiencing. For example, a specific display of stones is chosen to represent fear and, during a period of meditation, the patient reflects upon what is causing this fear, how it started, what makes it stronger or decreases it, in order to consciously work on strategies to overcome this feeling.

A previous case control blind assessment study conducted by our research group on patients with epilepsy suggested that "Mandalas of Emotion" may facilitate perception of feelings, since there was a significant difference between groups (Control, n = 20; Intervention, n = 26). There was a significant change in perception of emotion in the group that received Mandalas of Emotions. Moreover, the group that received intervention had significantly more perception of body changes and became more relaxed when compared to the control group.[16]

When compared to other techniques, like meditation, mindfulness, and acupuncture; mandalas of emotions present the advantage of being a low cost and non-invasive method that could be quickly and easily self-applied in any situation or place. In terms of cognitive demand for learning and training, application is easier than other methods like mindfulness and meditation. Mandalas are adaptable to different contexts, since there are different displays of stones in order to work on different emotions.

Thus, this technique presents immediate results in a sense that it allows individuals to act upon their emotions, and a long-term improvement in the ability to sustain self-care, since it empowers the person with straight-forward strategies to understand and cope with emotions. In this sense, we believe that the mandalas of emotions can represent a significant contribution to promoting self-care and copying during and after cancer treatment.

---

15   Ibid.
16   Ribeiro, Carolina, et al. "Mandala of Emotions facilitate perception of feelings" (paper presented at the annual meeting of the Brazilian Research Institute for Neuroscience and Neurotechnology, Campinas, Brazil, April 11–13th, 2016).

6   Final Reflections

This single case illustrates the use of ME as add-on therapy for self-healing and resolution of internal conflicts for a long period of time. Although the reported findings cannot be generalized, these results bring a perspective of a therapeutic potential for situations of emotional conflict, to promote self-understanding and healing, enabling the person to better cope with these emotions. Therefore, this case report provides useful preliminary evidence to an accumulating body of literature supporting the theory and efficacies of add-on techniques in cancer treatment.

7   The Last Take

The experience described above presented during the Global Conference "The Patient", at Mansfield College, University of Oxford, the UK, in September, 2016, was shared with the patient. She was in the final stage of cancer, and in one of the last visits with Dr. Ling, in October 2016, before passing away in the following week, the patient was lucid and described her views on the overall experience with Mandalas of Emotions and living with cancer treatment, as follows (our translation):

> [During the final stage] my oncologist allowed me to stay home and to clinically follow-up my blood exams and platelets levels once every two weeks. My body no longer allows me to perform daily activities such as going to the supermarket or driving. But the main issue is emotional. I am constantly afraid that the pain may return, and, at those times when I need to go to the hospital, I fear the pain that the treatment may inflict on me. Mandalas of emotions is helping me to cope with this fear. I use the mandalas when I wake up and before going to bed. It is the kind of therapy, of self-healing tool, I need at this moment.

8   Acknowledgements

This work was analysed at the Brazilian Research Institute for Neuroscience and Neurotechnology (BRAINN) one of the Research, Innovation and Dissemination Centers (RFID) supported by the São Paulo Research Foundation, as part of a research initiative in Chinese Medicine.

Bibliography

Kanavos, Panos. "The rising burden of cancer in the developing world." *Annals of Oncology* 17 (2006): 15–23.

Langley, Keith. "The Neuroendocrine Concept Today." *Annals of the New York Academy of Sciences* 733 (1994): 1–17.

Ling, Li Hui. *Dialogando com as emoções e promovendo a saúde.* Curitiba: Insight, 2013.

Ma, Xiaomei and Herbert Yu Ma. "Global Burden of Cancer." *Yale Journal of Biology and Medicine* 79 (2006): 85–94.

Miller, Kimberly D., Rebecca L. Siegel and Ahmedin Jemal. "Cancer statistics 2016." *CA: A Cancer Journal for Clinicians* 66 (2016): 271–289.

Öberg, Kjell and Daniel Castellano. "Current knowledge on diagnosis and staging of neuroendocrine tumors." *Cancer and Metastasis Reviews* 30 (2011): 3–7.

Ribeiro, Carolina, Li Hui Ling, Gabriela Salim Spagnol, Jéssica Elias Vicentini, Paula C.F. Oliveira and Li Min Li. "Mandala of Emotions facilitate perception of feelings." Paper presented at the annual meeting of the Brazilian Research Institute for Neuroscience and Neurotechnology, Campinas, Brazil, April 11-13th, 2016.

Sloan, Frank A. and Hellen Gelband. *Cancer control opportunities in low- and middle-income countries.* Washington, DC: National Academies Press, 2007.

CHAPTER 4

"Dialogue with Emotions" through the Eyes of Patients with Epilepsy and Caregivers

Gabriela Salim Spagnol, Jéssica Elias Vicentini, Isilda Sueli Andreolli Mira de Assumpção, Li Hui Ling and Li Li Min

1   Introduction

Epilepsy is a leading neurological disorder worldwide, with a rate prevalence of between 4 and 10 per 1000 people in developed countries and between 7 and 14 per 1,000 people in low– and middle-income countries. The proportions in these limited income countries constitute nearly 80% of the 70 million people worldwide with this condition.[1] In Brazil, there are approximately three million people with epilepsy, and to this number are added 300 new cases per day.[2]

Epilepsy is operationally defined as two or more unprovoked seizures occurring at least 24h apart,[3] or an underlying cause with an increased chance of seizure occurrence.[4] This disorder is characterized by unpredictable recurrent seizures, which can vary in frequency.[5] Seizures are described as brief episodes of involuntary movement that may reflect temporary dysfunction of specific neurons (focal seizures) or of a wider area involving both cerebral hemispheres (generalized seizures).[6]

Approximately 70% of people with epilepsy can control their seizures if given the appropriate medical treatment. Nevertheless, the burden of epilepsy can be substantial and complex, resulting in challenges in autonomy with a large weight in the psychological, physical, social and economic aspects,

1   Savvas Hadjikoutis, et al, "Approach to the patient with epilepsy in the outpatient department," *Postgraduate Medical Journal* 81 (2005): 442–447.
2   Ana L.A. Noronha, et al., "Prevalence and Pattern of Epilepsy Treatment in Different Socio-economic Classes in Brazil," *Epilepsia* 48 (2007): 880–885.
3   Commission on Epidemiology and Prognosis, International League Against Epilepsy, "Guidelines for epidemiologic studies on epilepsy," *Epilepsia* 34 (1993): 592–596.
4   Robert S. Fisher, et al., "ILAE Official Report: A practical clinical definition of epilepsy," *Epilepsia* 55(2014): 475–482.
5   Mary Jane England, et al., *Epilepsy across the spectrum: promoting health and understanding*, (Washington, DC: National Academies Press, 2012), 25–110.
6   Carlos A. M. Guerreiro, et al., *Epilepsia* (São Paulo: Lemos, 2000), 1–10.

© KONINKLIJKE BRILL NV, LEIDEN, 2019 | DOI:10.1163/9789004386563_006

revealing difficulties not only for the patient, but also for his or her family. This has ultimately consequences either in school, work or social environments.[7] At the time of diagnosis, patients and relatives face uncertainties, which rise from the lack of knowledge, beliefs, stigma, and fear of discrimination.[8] When these issues are not properly addressed, they can lead to poor self-esteem in patients, restrictions, and overprotection from the caregivers.[9] Quality of life is poorer in people suffering from epilepsy compared to the general population, and there is reportedly a higher prevalence of comorbidities.[10]

According to a survey on stigma in epilepsy,[11] social inclusion has been defined to be a major problem, since only half of the patients considered themselves socially engaged. This number probably reflects the rate of patients free of seizures, knowing that patients suffering frequent seizures have lower chances of professional or academic engagement. Furthermore, psychosocial issues and prejudice about epilepsy are one of the biggest barriers faced by patients, especially during school life and later at work.[12]

Over the past decades, patients, families and health professionals have gathered in non-governmental associations and organizations in order to guarantee the rights and social inclusion of those with epilepsy, playing an important role in the support of people with epilepsy in the fight against prejudice. These organizations are able to articulate public policies to capture the needs of patients related not only to medical care, but also to the social and economic aspects of their lives.

As beliefs and myths about the disease perpetuate stigma, projects and campaigns such as "Epilepsy Out of the Shadows" under the auspice of the World Health Organization (WHO), the International League Against Epilepsy (ILAE), the International Bureau for Epilepsy (IBE), as well as the Purple Day sponsored by Anita Kauffman Foundation – play a crucial role in disseminating knowledge about epilepsy, in order to reduce stigma and prejudice. These

7   Peter M. Bradley and Bruce Lindsay, "Care delivery and self-management strategies for adults with epilepsy," *Cochrane Database Systematic Review* 23(2008): 1–7.
8   Juliana Caixeta, et al., "Epilepsy perception amongst university students: a survey," *Arquivos de Neuro-Psiquiatria*, 65 (2007): 43–48.
9   Noelene Weatherby-Fell, "Epilepsy and media: implications for those whose role is to educate," *Ethical Human Psychology Psychiatry*, 13 (2011): 134–148; Bruce P. Hermann, et al., "A comparison of health-related quality of life in patients with epilepsy, diabetes and multiple sclerosis," *Epilepsy Research* 25 (1996): 113–118.
10   Ibid.
11   Paula T. Fernandes, et al., "Stigma scale of epilepsy: validation process," *Arquivos de Neuro-Psiquiatria*, 65 (2007): 35–42.
12   Paula T. Fernandes, et al., "Teachers perception about epilepsy," *Arquivos de Neuro-Psiquiatria*, 65 (2007): 28–34.

initiatives also show the importance of patient engagement in narrating their stories of how to overcome prejudice and challenges. In this sense, the Purple Day – an international grassroots effort dedicated to increasing awareness about epilepsy worldwide – was motivated by a nine years old girl's own struggles with epilepsy.

In 2008, this girl, called Cassidy Megan, wrote a letter to the International Bureau of Epilepsy and The International League Against Epilepsy describing that when she was diagnosed with epilepsy, she felt scared, embarrassed and alone, since she thought she was the only kid with epilepsy.[13] She kept it a secret, afraid of what others might think. One year later, the Epilepsy Association of Nova Scotia paid a visit to her school to teach about epilepsy. She noticed her friends wanted to learn more. When they asked the presenter if she knew anyone with epilepsy, she told them yes. That was when Cassidy told her mom and teacher that they could reveal to people that she also had epilepsy. She was still scared, but knew she would have the support of her classmates. Cassidy's goal in creating the Purple Day is to get people talking about epilepsy in an effort to dispel myths and inform those with seizures that they are not alone. The Epilepsy Association of Nova Scotia came on board in 2008 to help develop Cassidy's idea which is now known as the Purple Day for epilepsy campaign. She chose the colour purple referring to lavender and the day March 26th as the landmark of epilepsy awareness. Today, the Purple Day has become an international movement – also celebrated in Brazil, during which stories of patients with epilepsy are shared and disseminated.

In the late 1990s, the concept of Narrative Medicine arose, established, among others, by Rita Charon. This concept holds that medical practice focused on patient should include "stories of illness" in order to understand the personal experience regarding the disease.[14] The systematic record and analysis of patient stories is one of the approaches to promote the learning of students and physicians. Thus, this study applies this concept to contribute in professional education, and especially to disseminate knowledge and break down prejudice.

Since the high prevalence and incidence of stigma perceived by the individual with epilepsy may negatively affect health-related behaviours, including treatment, coping, and self-management and the psychosocial difficulties affect not only patients, but also family members, this study aimed at establishing

---

13   Cassidy Megan, letter from author to the members of the International Bureau of Epilepsy and The International League Against Epilepsy, 31 January 2014.

14   Rita Charon, *Narrative Medicine: honouring the stories of illness* (Oxford: Oxford University Press, 2006), 250–288.

a group for patients and caregivers with healthcare professionals, in order to promote psychosocial support and exchange of experiences.[15] Based on previous successful initiatives in the fight against stigma in epilepsy, afterwards, the record of these meetings was transcribed, analysed and converted into articles and books to disseminate knowledge about epilepsy.

2   Methods

We observed that patients arrived at least one hour ahead of medical consultation time. For this reason, the group session was planned to take place during this period, adding value to the patient during his or her stay at the hospital. This weekly group session lasted one hour, with approximately ten participants per session, and meetings were held for one year. This study was approved by the local Ethics Committee.

Patients, family and caregivers were invited to join the group, and also to contribute in this research, by signing a consent form, after it had been explained that sessions would be recorded. Participation in the group was allowed even without the contribution of a volunteer in this study. This meant that excerpts from transcripts with the volunteer contributions would be excluded from our records. However, all those who were invited to participate in the group were also keen on contributing in the research and signed the consent form.

Regarding ethical concerns, this study did not present risks to volunteers, nor did it provide any direct benefits to participants. However, it presented social benefits, since we infer that a better understanding regarding the life of a person with epilepsy may help understand the difficulties and limitations of this disease, and also help motivate participants when listening to stories about clinical improvements and quality of life. All recordings remained confidential and anonymous.

3   Results

After each group session, recordings were transcribed and later analysed. They were grouped in themes as per their frequency of report.

---

15   Emily B. Leaffer, et al., "Psychosocial and sociodemographic associates of felt stigma in epilepsy," *Epilepsy Behaviour* 37 (2014): 104–109.

A   *Fear, Shame and Lack of Control*

This feeling was reported by patients in relation to several situations:

– Shame/fear of suffering from a seizure in a public place:

> In the beginning, I used to be terrified of having a seizure in public, as I had in the market once. Those around me warned the entire market, and lots of people surrounded me – when I woke up I saw them looking at me. So it was really embarrassing and I was always afraid of experiencing this situation again.

– Shame/fear of losing consciousness and control of bowel or bladder function during a seizure:

> I was stirring a pot on the stove, when I realized that I was not okay. A few seconds later, I tried to sit down, to lean on something. By the time I came back to my senses, my hand was holding the sink and the carpet was wet. I had had urine loss. I went outside to quickly wash the carpet ... and I started to wonder ... what had happened?

– Shame/fear of telling family members, friends, classmates and co-workers about epilepsy;
– Fear of not being able to carry out or keep a job;
– Fear/shame of not being able to work or perform specific tasks, nor to carry out daily activities such as self-care and cooking without assistance.

B   *Restriction and Adaptation*

Patients often reported a feeling of limitation and of being "prisoners," as seen in this excerpt, followed by an adaptation phase:

> I have always had my independence, I could go anywhere, work, and all the sudden [after epilepsy was diagnosed], I lost this freedom. Sometimes I go out without letting people know, because I was feeling trapped. What kind of life will I be able to live? Will I be able to do anything I like? It is like I said earlier, I don't want to stay home, I get bored easily, so I look for something to do, then it [the restriction after epilepsy was diagnosed] was a shock. Sometimes I have stupid thoughts in my mind, but after a couple of days, I start to realize that I am actually still able to do some things [related to leisure, cooking and daily activities]. – patient A.

C   *Stigma and Prejudice*

Patients and family narrated stories concerning the interpersonal relationships in social environments, such as school, the workplace and the home,
where stigma and prejudice were expressed verbally or in attitudes that could
culminated in social isolation for those with epilepsy.

D   *Lack of Knowledge*

Participants posed questions that showed gaps in their knowledge concerning:
- The etiology and pathophysiology of epilepsy;
- The process of clinical diagnosis and importance of exams such as electro-
  encephalogram, telemetry and magnetic resonance;
- How to proceed during a seizure;
- Different types of seizure and how to identify them;
- About the surgery: patients reported fear to submit to the surgery since they
  did not understand the procedure and they had false expectations con-
  cerning outcomes after surgery, such as no need to continue medication
  treatment.

These questions were either responded by a healthcare professional (nurse
or psychologist) or by other patients and participants, who had successful life
experiences and knowledge to share.

E   *Medication Compliance*

Medication compliance refers to whether patients take their medications as
prescribed and to whether they continue to take a prescribed medication. Stories reflected serious misconceptions about the treatment, such as the idea
that in the absence of a crisis, medication could be suspended, but effective
strategies to sustain the treatment were also reported, such as visual reminders
and association of the medication schedule with meals provided to prevent
lapses.

F   *Safety*

Strategies to continue activities at work, in the leisure time and/or at home
without compromising safety (I), as well as practices to decrease exposure to
seizure triggers (II):

> I – 'We [*patient A's family*] have never forbidden him to go out. Some-
> times he has a seizure in a public place, but people already know him
> and help him out. There is also a very dangerous staircase at our home, so
> we ask him not to climb it without supervision, and we asked him not to
> drive anymore, because it is not safe' – *patient A's son.*

II – 'I met a guy who could not go to night clubs [*because of light shows that are seizure triggers*]. I realized that when he had little sleep or when he drank too much coffee, he had more seizures. So he changed his habits'.

G   *Memory Deficits, Especially after Seizures*

It is a strange thing [*waking up after a seizure*]. On my daughter's wedding, I could not remember how I had arrived at the venue. I only remember her with a piece of handkerchief drying my lips. I remember we were on a familiar road, and I thought I was okay. But I was having a seizure.

3   Discussion

A   *Fear, Shame and Lack of Control*

Fear and shame can precede any situation of discrimination and become common in daily living with epilepsy and commonly evolve into behavioural changes (shame, insecurity, isolation) and greater difficulties in psychosocial adjustment.[16] In our study, these emotions were mostly related to the seizure, restrictions that epilepsy may have on daily activities and the prejudice one may face when sharing with others about epilepsy. These attitudes are reinforced by lack of knowledge and prejudice. Public education can change perceptions, and consequently, lead to greater social acceptance of those with epilepsy.

B   *Restriction and Adaptation*

Patients in our study reported that epilepsy and its treatment implied restrictions and adaptations in their daily lives. Several studies describe that epilepsy impacts on relationships, social life, employment, and plans for the future.[17] In our study, most narratives depicted a scenario in which patients and family members followed a similar route: after receiving the diagnosis of epilepsy and

---

16   Fernandes, et al., "Stigma scale of epilepsy: validation process," 35–42.
17   Gus A. Baker, et al., "Quality of life of people with epilepsy: a European study" *Epilepsia* 38 (1997): 353–362; Ann Jacoby, et al., "Public knowledge, private grief: a study of public attitudes to epilepsy in the United Kingdom and implications for stigma," *Epilepsia* 45 (2004): 1405–1415; Marju Herodes, et al., "Epilepsy in Estonia: a quality-of-life study" *Epilepsia* 42 (2001): 1061–1073; Arthur Kleinman, et al., "The social course of epilepsy: chronic illness as social experience in interior China," *Social Sciences Medicine* 40 (1995): 1319–1330.

its treatment there was a general feeling of restriction and fear related to the new life conditions. But the following experiences also lead to new possibilities, mutual support and resilience to adapt, in order to pursue welfare for patients suffering from epilepsy and personal fulfilment.

C   Stigma and Prejudice

When it comes to psychosocial difficulties, stigma is the first aspect to be addressed. According to Goffman (1963),[18] the stigmatized person is considered to be having different characteristics and receives a different treatment by the community, which assumes prejudiced concepts in relation to this particular person. It is an aspect which influences the person's health in a global way, including their physical and psychological well-being.

A study by Fernandes and colleagues[19] described a negative correlation between level of education (illiterate to higher education) and stigma score in Brazil, in which as the level of education rises, the perception of stigma decreases. The same pattern was described for socioeconomic classes, suggesting that lack of knowledge is one aspect of stigma, since information access increases according to educational and socioeconomic level. However, another possibility is that people may have offered "politically correct" answers. Also in this study, an unexpected finding was the difference in level of epilepsy stigma between women and men, with women demonstrating higher stigma perception.

Misconceptions about epilepsy are still common and, in some cases, may imply superstitious perceptions, such as the belief that epilepsy is "God's punishment." In this sense, Fernandes and colleagues state that the perception of epilepsy is influenced by each person's beliefs, particularly by the religious faith.[20] When comparing different religious groups, Fernandes and colleagues[21] observed the lowest scores for those who declared an affiliation with Spiritism, which is a doctrine based on belief in superior spirits and communication with these spirits through a medium.

D   Lack of Knowledge

Seizure control is the starting point but not sufficient to ensure a normal life for these patients. When compared to people without epilepsy, patients with

---

18   Erving Goffman, *Stigma: notes on the management of spoiled identity.* (New York: Touchstone, 1963), 10–25.

19   Fernandes, et al., "Stigma scale of epilepsy: validation process," 35–42.

20   Ibid.

21   Ibid.

epilepsy appear to have a very different life, because they suffer greater social isolation, greater difficulty in social relationships, and higher unemployment rates, among others. It is important that people know what epilepsy is, what it implies, and what the psychological difficulties are, in order to decrease the burden of prejudice inflicted upon the patient and his/her family. In this context, we created the group dialoguing with the emotions, in order to give support to people with epilepsy, by promoting personal resilience, improved quality of life, and sharing emotions and experiences.[22]

E   *Medication Compliance*

The available treatment that relies on the correct use of antiepileptic medication can control epilepsies in 70% of cases with a single drug, and, in 10% of cases, if medications are combined. Results of a systematic review of the literature by Meyer and colleagues suggest that there are dramatic global disparities in the care and treatment of epilepsy patients.[23] The reasons for this non-treatment are complex, and include: the wish for non-treatment, lack of knowledge about an existing treatment, an unprepared health system to treat the patients, and social stigma. In this sense, it is necessary to follow the hierarchy of care: low complexity epilepsy should be treated in primary care, and high complexity epilepsy in tertiary centres, where treatment plans could rely on a combination of drugs, new therapies, and surgical treatment.

F   *Safety*

In Campinas, a city of one million people and with universal access to health care, the treatment gap (patient untreated or inappropriate medication regime) of people with epilepsy is 40%.[24] This means that almost half of the people with epilepsy are unprotected from the risk of injury or death as a result of crises. People with epilepsy need the support of those around them to secure safety conditions to sustain their daily activities at home, school and work.

G   *Memory Deficits*

Memory deficit is one of the most common symptoms after seizures. As highlighted in the previous section, those surrounding people with epilepsy must

---

22   Humberto Maturana, *Ontology Reality* (Belo Horizonte: UFMG, 1997), 167–181.

23   England, et al., "Epilepsy across the spectrum: promoting health and understanding," 25–110.

24   Noronha, et al., "Prevalence and Pattern of Epilepsy Treatment in Different Socioeconomic Classes in Brazil," 880–885.

be sensible enough to provide not only safety precautions but also emotional support after seizures have occurred.

4   Conclusion

During these meetings, patients, family members and caregivers could exchange information and advice others to learn about epilepsy and its management, providing sympathetic understanding. Close friends and family showed engagement in sharing their experiences, providing support to deal with issues related to epilepsy. Further explanation on specific topics was covered by healthcare professionals, who demystified and clarified misconceptions and also mediated the group dynamic.

Sharing patient stories allows for making sense of their suffering and how it feels from the inside. Sharing stories offers a biographic and social context of the illness experience and suggests coping strategies, creating potential for personal development. In this sense, "Dialogue with Emotions" can be an alternative way for patients and families living with epilepsy to discuss and share their feelings. This is the first step in the process towards overcoming barriers and improving quality of life. In this setting, patients and caregivers are at same level as healthcare professionals, who empower and encourage patients to seek his/her own solution and ability to understand epilepsy.

Bibliography

Baker, Gus A., Ann Jacoby, Deborah Buck, Carlos Stalgis and Dominique Monnet. "Quality of life of people with epilepsy: a European study." *Epilepsia* 38 (1997): 353–362.

Bradley, Peter M. and Bruce Lindsay. Care delivery and self-management strategies for adults with epilepsy. *Cochrane Database Syst Rev*, 23 (2008): 1–7.

Bruce P. Hermann, Barbara Vickrey, Ron D. Hays, Joyce Cramer, Orrin Devinsky, Kimford Meador, Kenneth Perrine, Lawrence W. Myers and George W. Ellison. "A comparison of health-related quality of life in patients with epilepsy, diabetes and multiple sclerosis." *Epilepsy Research* 25 (1996): 113–118.

Caixeta, Juliana, Paula T. Fernandes, Gail S. Bell, Josemir W. Sander and Li Min Li. "Epilepsy perception amongst university students: a survey." *Arquivos de Neuro-Psiquiatria*, 65 (2007): 43–48.

Charon, Rita. *Narrative Medicine: honouring the stories of illness*. Oxford: Oxford University Press, 2006.

Commission on Epidemiology and Prognosis, International League Against Epilepsy. "Guidelines for epidemiologic studies on epilepsy." *Epilepsia* 34 (1993): 592–596.

England, Mary Jane, Catharyn T Liverman, Andrea M Schultz and Larisa M Strawbridge. *Epilepsy across the spectrum: promoting health and understanding.* Washington, DC: National Academies Press, 2012.

Fernandes, Paula T., Ana L.A. Noronha, Ulisses Araújo, Paula Cabral, Ricardo Pataro and Hanneke M. de Boer. "Teachers perception about epilepsy." *Arquivos de Neuro-Psiquiatria*, 65 (2007): 28–34.

Fernandes, Paula T., Priscila C.B. Salgado, Ana L.A. Noronha, Josemir W. Sander and Li Min Li. "Stigma scale of epilepsy: validation process." *Arquivos de Neuro-Psiquiatria*, 65 (2007): 35–42.

Fisher, Robert S., Carlos Acevedo, Alexis Arzimanoglou, Alicia Bogacz, J. Helen Cross, Christian E. Elger, Jerome Engel Jr, Lars Forsgren, Jacqueline A. French, Mike Glynn, Dale C. Hesdorffer, B.I. Lee, Gary W. Mathern, Solomon L. Moshé, Emilio Perucca, Ingrid E. Scheffer, Torbjörn Tomson, Masako Watanabe, Samuel Wiebe. "ILAE Official Report: A practical clinical definition of epilepsy." *Epilepsia* 55(2014): 475–482.

Goffman, Erving. *Stigma: notes on the management of spoiled identity.* New York: Touchstone, 1963.

Guerreiro, Carlos A. M., Marilisa M. Guerreiro, Fernando Cendes and Íscia Lopes-Cendes. *Epilepsia.* São Paulo: Lemos, 2000.

Hadjikoutis, Savvas and Philip E. M. Smith. "Approach to the patient with epilepsy in the outpatient department." *Postgraduate Medical Journal* 81 (2005): 442–447.

Herodes, Marju, Andre Õun, Sulev Haldre and Ain-Elmar Kaasik. "Epilepsy in Estonia: a quality-of-life study." *Epilepsia* 42 (2001): 1061–1073.

Jacoby, Ann, Joanne Gorry, Carrol Gamble and Gus A. Baker. "Public knowledge, private grief: a study of public attitudes to epilepsy in the United Kingdom and implications for stigma." *Epilepsia* 45 (2004):1405–1415.

Kleinman, Arthur, Wen-Zhi Wang, Shi-Chuo Li, Xue-Ming Cheng, Xiu-Ying Dai, Kun-Tun Li and Joan Kleinman. "The social course of epilepsy: chronic illness as social experience in interior China." *Social Sciences Medicine* 40 (1995): 1319–1330.

Leaffer, Emily B., Dale C. Hesdorffer, Charles Begley E.B. Leaffer, D.C. Hesdorffer and C. Begley. "Psychosocial and sociodemographic associates of felt stigma in epilepsy." *Epilepsy Behaviour* 37 (2014): 104–109.

Maturana, Humberto. *Ontology Reality.* Belo Horizonte: UFMG, 1997.

Noronha, Ana L.A., Moacir A. Borges, Lucia H.N. Marques, Dirce M.T. Zanetta, Paula T. Fernandes, Hanneke M. de Boer, Javier Espíndola, Claudio T. Miranda, Leonid Prilipko, Gail S. Bell, Josemir W. Sander and Li Min Li. "Prevalence and Pattern of Epilepsy Treatment in Different Socioeconomic Classes in Brazil." *Epilepsia* 48 (2007): 880–885.

Weatherby-Fell, Noelene. "Epilepsy and media: implications for those whose role is to educate." *Ethical Human Psychology Psychiatry*, 13 (2011).

CHAPTER 5

Self-Understanding and Self-Healing

Sônia Aparecida Bortolotto Torezan

1   My Story[1]

The life of God the Father flows into us. As we breathe, we are grant-ed health and strength. We are happy and we feel better each and every day. Vibrations of peace and harmony destined to all beings in the universe come from our minds and our hearts. We are fine, our thoughts are with God. He quiets our hearts, protects our health and renews our healthy cells. We are immune, averse and refractory to negative thoughts, words and actions. Everything good will come to us at the right time. We had cancer and other serious diseases. We are now in a self-healing process and we feel fine.[2]

My story began in February, 2014, when I was diagnosed with melanoma, after the analysis of a skin mole on my left arm. After that I underwent tests to see if there were other outbreaks and prepared for surgery to remove the mole.

When that happened, I was attending a post-graduation program at an im-portant university in the state of Minas Gerais (I live in the state of São Paulo), worked as a social worker in the city where I live, and twice a week I worked as a professor at a private college in a neighbouring town. I was forced to stop all my professional activities.

---

1 'After doing everything in her power to fight the disease, Sônia passed away on June 10th, 2018. She lived 57 full years and leaves husband and two sons. She was a dear and loyal family member and friend, who was present in very many details of the lives she touched, also as a colleague and as a public agent. She helped very many people and will always be remem-bered by her bright eyes, easy smile and energy to find solutions to our hardships in life. As a researcher and social worker, she defended young adults and children against social and family violence, showing the importance of art workshop practices for those in assisted free-dom (available at http://repositorio.unicamp.br/jspui/handle/REPOSIP/252914). She will be deeply missed.' – Davina Marques, June 12, 2018.

2 This is a 'mantra' of unknown authorship. I was taught by a very dear friend of mine who underwent surgery in 1988, for being diagnosed with cancer. I have changed it to suit my own thoughts.

The surgery took place on April 30, 2014, and soon after I regained consciousness after the anaesthesia the doctor came to my room and informed me that the biopsy had come back as positive for melanoma also in two lymph nodes, and as a result it was necessary to empty my armpit. I went home in a lot of pain, with a drain for blood and difficulties to lie down, to get around and perform basic daily activities. When the bandage on my left arm was removed for the first time, I was able to check the size of the mutilation I had suffered in order to reduce the risk of leaving a cancerous cell behind.

In oncology centres all over the world, there are thousands, millions of people with all kinds of mutilations. The first indication for the treatment of cancer is extirpating, tearing, cutting off the affected area or organ. This causes a multitude of people who, just like war veterans, have their bodies mutilated, opened up and stitched; their faces transfigured, with no guarantees that they will be cured. In medicine, a doctor told me, it is unethical to tell a patient that he or she will be cured.

The cancer patient faces the stigma of society when the physical changes are easily seen: one becomes bald; there are no eyebrows; lesions show on one's face, head and limbs. Other deformities may be hidden, like severed breasts, surgery scars, radiation therapy burns, and scars. However, in intimacy they are visible and the person may be shaken in his/her self-esteem.

When we talk about cancer, however, mutilation and vanity are the smallest of the worries. It is a matter of life and death and the efforts are to terminate, to end the problem; it is not a cosmetic issue. The surgeon who operated on me said 'I did what had to be done.' He was at that point more worried with the result of the biopsy of the other lymph nodes that he had removed. When the results showed that both the removed lymph nodes and the tissue were negative for melanoma, this was a great relief.

This, however, was nothing but a temporary relief: treatment is required to try to prevent new occurrences of cancer or the infamous metastases. In my case, the possibilities were no further treatments and only controls through CT scans, or undergoing Interferon treatment, a medication which is more effective for cases of hepatitis C. This second option was recommended by my doctor.

Despite having received information about the very harmful body reactions with Interferon intake, and even its little efficacy, I opted for this treatment. While using this medication, there were changes in my breast lymph nodes (mediastinum) and a new surgery was scheduled to remove them. The biopsy showed I had developed a disease called sarcoidosis. I opted for the interruption of this treatment after six months of use and before the twelve-month ideal time span.

From February to September, 2015, I was not subjected to any treatment, and then my chest tomography displayed a nodule in the left lung, which required removal through surgery. The biopsy result: melanoma metastases in the lungs.

This diagnosis messed with my self-control and disturbed the certainty of healing that I had gradually started to gain. I was in a new denial phase: 'They have mismanaged my exams, I have nothing, I feel no pain, it is a big mistake and I'll wake up from this nightmare!' In December, 2015, I was affected by a state of melancholy and sadness that prevented me from embarking in January to Peru with dear friends and visit Machu Picchu. I had no courage to face people because I felt guilty for being in this situation of disease.

Concurrently with the allopathic medical treatment, I had started acupuncture, yoga, and Ayurveda therapy with an emphasis on nutrition and a meditation group once a week. Between December and January, I met a Jin Shin Jyutsu professional, who worked with me and taught me techniques to do exercises at home. These gave me the balance back and reduced the symptoms of sadness and melancholy.

I was afraid of dying! For the first time and intensely, I was affected by concrete thoughts about the finiteness of life. I was not in possession of the results of a PET scan, from December, and when I met my oncologist I was told that there were several points of metastases in my body, with the characteristic of being subcutaneous. I was given another treatment, now with Vermurafenib. Some of the side effects I experienced were joint pain, nausea, and malaise. The first major reaction occurred thirteen days after I started the treatment: a rash covered most of my body, with the exception of my face and neck. My dermatologist demanded the interruption of the medication, because she feared it would lead me to Stevens Johnson Syndrome. This possibility was later discarded, as I treated the rash with corticosteroids.

I reduced the daily dose of Vermurafenib from eight to six tablets. There were other reactions: joint pain (arthritis, carpal tunnel syndrome), skin reactions (thick skin with lots of warts and moles, some of which were taken for analysis), and finally the drug triggered the hair and eyebrow to fall off.

At this stage I started to show signs of acceptance, I started reading about miracles and extraordinary cures (as one of the books suggested in its title). These were successive cycles and they emerged sequentially and naturally.

2   Alternative Practices and Spirituality

Many people had told me about cures performed through an internationally known medium: João de Deus (John of God). I went to the city where he lives,

Abadiania, in the central Brazilian state of Goiás. There I got involved with his healing by entities; many of these were doctors whose lives had been dedicated to spiritualism. The trips to João de Deus were in groups and conducted by guides.

I've been to Abadiania four times. The first two were with one guide and the last two with another. I consider this second guide an inspiration and an example of a journey of self-healing. G. was diagnosed with breast cancer at the age of 35 and had a mastectomy (breast removal) followed by all the indicated treatment until the tests results led to the diagnosis that she was considered cured. Two years later, after feeling deep pain, further tests revealed that the cancer had returned, in the bones. In 2013 she received the 'sentence' that she only had six more months to live. She was in real pain at that stage and ended up in a wheelchair. G.'s aunt had been to Abadiania and had given her name to the medium João de Deus, who prescribed her the medication prepared at Casa Dom Inácio, where he works. These drugs are passionflower tablets. As one consults the medium, the entity that he has incorporated spiritually adds in the remedy that the person needs in order to get better or heal.

G. received the passionflower from her aunt and started taking it. She started getting better, left the wheelchair and was feeling so good that she decided to meet the medium João de Deus. Since then, for nearly three years now, she has been going monthly to Abadiania. Because news travels fast, people began to go to Abadiania with G. as a guide. Her PET scan shows that she still has stains of bone metastases, but these have decreased significantly without chemotherapy. Doctors say it is a true miracle, because she does not feel any pain, she shows vitality and performs her daily activities normally.

When my PET scan showed metastases I met G. through Ayurveda and the fact that I was in contact with a person with metastases who was alive and feeling well gave me a lot of strength and hope. I do not know how I would have survived the result of these exams if I had not met G..

Despite all the battle strength of cancer patients, living with the certainty of this disease brings an instability that makes us very vulnerable. We are in a constant state of alert that often prevents us from enjoying complete moments of happiness. G. says that when you wake up in the morning, you feel like you have a gun pointed at your face.

As I write this paper, I receive the news that my friend G. met an entity incorporated by João de Deus, who told her she was cured. It is a great joy and perhaps many might say that this being cured does not make much sense, but for those of us who know him, who are involved with his deeds and we have seen the thousands of healings that take place in Abadiania, it has a great and definitive meaning. He does not tell someone that she is cured randomly or per se. We know that, when he says that, it is because the person was blessed with healing, and she has earned it.

Another event in my journey of spirituality was meeting Alice, a healer. This lady was born in Paraguaçu, in the Brazilian state of Minas Gerais, where her family has a piece of farm land in which Our Lady of Aparecida appears. Mrs. Alice says she has seen and talked to Our Lady for over twenty years, and at her request a grotto with her image was built.

At this place, ribbons are attached to the hand of the image of the Lady and people hold its other end. Mrs. Alice, usually around noon, stands in front of the image and Our Lady tells her what the person holding the tape should do to heal. She is consulted on other matters as well, such as the behaviour of loved ones, labour and financial situations. There is a water spring in the grotto and people collect it in bottles to drink and to wash the affected areas of the body as a form of treatment. Water can be increased at certain times of the day and one's mission consists of praying by using a rosary and praying to Our Lady of Aparecida over a certain number of days.

Mrs. Alice, though illiterate, keeps books of accounts of numerous people who received healings and graces; these are written by the very people who were honoured, along with photos of the state of people before and after healing. Her own account was the grace to have had her daughter born healthy, when doctors said the child would not be born alive. Faith, according to Mrs. Alice, is clear and unquestionable. In her simplicity she says she talks to Our Lady and gives people Her message.

In my case, since the first time I met Mrs. Alice, the message of Our Lady was that I can heal. The most impressive is that she knew that I took very strong drugs. She says I take the medicine to fix one thing and that it is bad for others. When she meets someone, Mrs. Alice says assertive things about some treatments. With regard to mine, she always says: 'how much money is being spent on your treatment.'

This leads me to reflect upon medicine and the pharmaceutical industry, the high cost of tests and treatments to treat and try to cure cancer, and how many of them are nothing but palliative! Vermurafenib, according to my oncologist, is palliative. You take it and the lumps are gone; you stop taking them, and the lumps are back. According to this perspective, the patient with melanoma metastases should take Vermurafenib or any other market drug for the rest of his/her days. It makes us wonder that this 'lifetime' for melanoma carrier are not many days/months; they talk of 'survival expectancy.'

We are confused when we hear that there is already a cure for cancer and it is not revealed because it would end the profits of big business of this branch.

Could that be true? In this perverse system, being the patient in a weakened state is just more aggravating.

3   Alternative Treatments: Ayurveda

Ayurveda has taught me, among other things, about meditation. I have meditated weekly, in group. We always start with a devotional chant, Samgacchadvam, to create a collective flow of energy before the group meditation. The song calls for a collaborative movement, irradiating the same thought and an invitation to enjoy the resources of the universe, just as the ancient sages did. It is a call to a common ideal, in order to inspire hearts and minds to be inseparable, hoping that we will be together as *One*.

One should meditate every day, in groups or alone, as this is part of an alternative practice to search for healing and health.

Besides the conventional medical treatment, I have sought to find treatments that make me believe and engage in working for a cure. A cancer patient who is tired of fighting dies! Every day is a struggle for maintaining physical and mental health. This is another kind of existence, based on perseverance and persistence. We could say that life hangs by a thread which is sustained by thoughts that must be positive.

When we learn of the deaths of people from cancer, we feel our perseverance in healing tremble. G. thinks differently, she reminds us that everyone will eventually die, many will even die before the cancer patients, so why torture ourselves?

While in medicine we may not hear the doctor say the words 'you have a cure,' in alternative practices therapists lead us to think that healing is within us. Consultations with the Ayurveda therapist make me happy; the professional approach is a personalized service where we are given time to be listened to and are told many things. It is not a maudlin language based on statements that give false hopes to the patient, but a treatment line with solid foundations, theoretically based in an ancient Indian culture.

The treatment in alternative practices requires the constant search for knowledge, belief in healing and in the capacity for self-healing, discipline, giving up many things that hitherto were important or good for us, and especially the courage to often say 'no' to a given medical treatment.

Spouses, children, and close friends believe that everything can go back to being the way they were before the surgery. A person who has had cancer will never be the same; in order to be healthy, even when living with the disease, one must radically change the diet, daily routines with exercises and meditation, among other practices, in a way that the patient designs for him/herself.

I see the positive aspects of this change because they lead to self-knowledge, better relationships with others, habits that provide health, vitality, and self-control. Another good thing is that this behaviour can be contagious and affect those around us, when they see their loved ones become better and believe that these practices are beneficial, trying to follow them as well.

The patient must not lose hope. Rather, harbouring the thought that life should be fully lived every day, one can dream and believe in miracles. The thought of a remaining lifetime or life expectancy for a patient with cancer leads to depression. If God alone can set the start and end day of people's lives, why then establish statistics on how much life lies ahead?

Alternative practices carried out along with the intake of chemotherapy lead the patient to a better quality of life, as they decrease the intensity of the reactions that these drugs cause the body. The ideal situation, however, is having these alternative practices as a daily routine in a cancer patient's life and achieving a cure, performing these activities regularly and with discipline.

In the narratives of patients with serious diseases, who were declared incurable by medicine but were still cured, the most significant and common factor is the thought and the belief in healing. Other factors that lead to healing according to these patients are exercises of all kinds; from yoga, hiking, fitness, Pilates, among others, a diet based on varied knowledge (of macrobiotics, Ayurveda, vegetarian etc.), the support from family and friends, religion and meditation. The fact that the patient believes and has no doubts that he/she will be cured materializes health.

CHAPTER 6

Presenting the Patient: through a Storytelling, Illness and Medicine Lens

Peter Bray

1 Introduction

As the event leader for both "Storytelling, Illness and Medicine" and "The Patient" conferences I was curious to analyse and understand the themes that emerged from the former and tie them into those that might be raised in our present conference. A significant and recurrent theme from the last "Patient"[1] conference suggested that the integrity of an individual's identity is "challenged by the experience of suffering,"[2] and previous conferences have also emphasised the "the social aspects of caring."[3] Whilst it is understood that this small sample of conference papers does not fully represent the field, this research identifies patient-related themes that emerged from our first "Storytelling, Illness and Medicine"[4] conference that speak into, and might further extend, discussions that arose in our current conference.[5]

2 Method

Using qualitative thematic analysis this small-scale study captures the ways in which conference participants represent the patient in their papers, and examines this patterned response within the data set.[6] It searches the conference's

---

1 The 4th Global Conference, "The Patient: Therapeutic Approaches," Prague, Czech Republic, 17th–19th March, 2014.
2 Peter Bray and Ana Borlescu, eds., "Introduction" *Beyond Present Patient Realities: Collaboration, Care and Identity* (Oxford, England: Inter-Disciplinary Press, 2015), xii.
3 Ibid., xiii
4 "The 6th Global Conference, Storytelling, Illness and Medicine," Budapest, Hungary, March 14–16, 2016 (SIM, 2016).
5 "The 5th Global Conference, The Patient: Examining Realities," Oxford, United Kingdom, 5th–7th September, 2016.
6 Virginia Braun and Victoria Clarke, "Using Thematic Analysis in Psychology" *Qualitative Research in Psychology* (2006): 78.

© KONINKLIJKE BRILL NV, LEIDEN, 2019 | DOI:10.1163/9789004386563_008

10 sessions and its 30 presentations to capture repeated patterns of meaning. The key conference themes are examined as well as those emerging themes that capture the essential ways in which patients are represented to provide an overall flavour of the conference experience. As the research approach is conducted within a constructionist framework, which examines "the effects of a range of discourses operating within society,"[7] and is driven by the analyst's theoretical interests, and the semantic content of the data, the work of developing these themes has involved a degree of interpretation.

3   Data Sources

Data for this analysis was drawn from four sources: abstracts and papers made available on the conference website; contemporaneous notes made by the researcher during the presentations of papers and expanded in discussions with delegates; papers resubmitted to the conference website after the conference to include material modified by the impact of the conference experience; notes made at the final development meeting where delegates discussed their ideas and themes for moving the project forward.

4   Themes and Analysis

Once the conference was over it was possible to be completely immersed in the four data sources and to identify ideas that might subsequently yield initial codes.[8] Data were systematically coded across the entire data set, and data collated relevant to each code. Codes were then sorted into broad themes and data gathered, and the sub-themes incorporated into the main themes. Finally, themes were reviewed to check their utility as both accurate and valid representations of the data set and to include any codes or themes missed from the initial phase.

The following analysis presents the main themes and, by way of example, their sub-themed constellations to not only provide a picture of the ways patients were presented by the conference but also to tell their own "story" of the event and its rich interdisciplinary discussions and learning.

---

7   Ibid., 81.
8   Ibid., 86–93. Six phases of thematic analysis.

A   *Health and the Person*

[Patients] have a need and a desire to share their stories ...[9]

As the obsession with health becomes a growing Western phenomenon and good health is regarded as a right, so tolerance of illness diminishes and ill-health is no longer seen as an inevitable flaw in the human condition. Recovery through natural means is the gold-standard of consumerised health which leaves conventional medical practice as a safe but less attractive intervention. Consequently, perceived as unnatural, fundamentally wrong, or even incoherent, modern medicine and Nature have become increasingly polarised. Thus, illness and disease remain synonymous with difference and its transformed host, no longer a passive victim, carries the responsibility for spreading instability and fear.[10] In this story the doctor and his medicine are represented as the only thing that stands between human order and chaos, whilst an aloof Nature looks on.

Alternatively, patients may also be depicted as consumers of health, refugees from a sick world seeking healthier lifestyles in natural environments, "islands of healing,"[11] and utopian communities. In this narrative mankind reveres Nature as an ideal state or context – Eden before the fall where illness is absent – a place of grace that human beings may return to and no longer be patients.

It is suggested that medicalising processes may also be responsible for making patients of groups that exhibit deviant or uncharacteristic behaviours that fail to conform to societal norms. This process further labels already vulnerable members of society, removes their agency and purposefully makes them more passive.[12] Such people have in the past been forcibly removed from society and themselves and placed in secure environments.[13]

---

9   Jane Youell, Alison Ward and Miranda Quinney, "Sharing Stories for Wellbeing," (paper presented at The 6th Global Conference, Storytelling, Illness and Medicine, Budapest, Hungary, March 2016).

10   Justyna Jajszczok, "The Stories of Invading Microbes: Infection Literature," (paper presented at The 6th Global Conference, Storytelling, Illness and Medicine, Budapest, Hungary, March 2016).

11   Silvia Carnelli, "Back to Eden in the 20th-century Europe: Monte Verità & Glastonbury. (Hi)Stories from two 'alternative' Isles of Healing," (paper presented at The 6th Global Conference, Storytelling, Illness and Medicine, Budapest, Hungary, March 2016).

12   Sofia Castanheira Pais, "From Normative to Deviant Behaviour: Health and Illness Definitions Related to Children and Adolescents' Perspectives," (paper presented at The 6th Global Conference, Storytelling, Illness and Medicine, Budapest, Hungary, March 2016).

13   Verusca Calabria, "Insider Stories from the Asylum: Exploring Peer and Staff-Patient Relationships," (paper presented at The 6th Global Conference, Storytelling, Illness and Medicine, Budapest, Hungary, March 2016).

The impact of illness is both personal and political. It is easy to assume that once people are diagnosed that they relinquish their aspirations and life's work to become their illness and withdraw into its othering lifestyle. Patients choose how to adapt to this new state either allowing it to shape their lives or by attempting to master it. Either way it becomes a powerful lens through which they now see the world. "Let us turn our pain to power, our victimhood to fire, our self-hatred to action, our self-obsession to service."[14] Broadly speaking patients were valued by the conference for their authenticity as individuals, groups and communities who, regardless of their very difficult circumstances, were able to share their journeys toward health, and offer empowering inspirational support to their families, caregivers, and other patients.

B   *The Patient, Research and Autoethnography*
      ... to construct a narrative that feels true to my experience.[15]

A small number of the participants disclosed their lived experiences as both a patient and a researcher managing difficult health issues:
      A visually impaired delegate suggested that, in representing the patient, we should not only be interested in what the world makes of disability but build a bridge into their "thoughtscape[s]"[16] – the unique, liminal and creative landscape of their inner existence.
      Wrestling with multiple interpretations concerning the truth of her condition, a young doctoral student recalls that her greatest hurdle was discovering how difficult it was to understand her "ambiguous and objectively unknown"[17] condition, whilst still being able to make major decisions about her health, "aware these decisions are based on a story that may or may not be correct."[18]
      A psychotherapist, describing her dark and choiceless journey into mental illness, also explained that it was like returning home. She suggested that although confrontation with the suffering self is feared, "cultural practices,

---

14   Marta Fernández-Morales, "In Me and Everywhere: Making Meaning of Cancer' citing Eve Ensler in Eve Ensler's memoir *In the Body of the World*," (paper presented at The 6th Global Conference, Storytelling, Illness and Medicine, Budapest, Hungary, March 2016).

15   Thembi Soddell, "Sound Experience: Listening Session and Discussion on the Experience of Invisible Illness," (paper presented at The 6th Global Conference, Storytelling, Illness and Medicine, Budapest, Hungary, March 2016).

16   Sandeep Singh, "Life-writing and the Disabled Self: Discourses on Subjectivity," (paper presented at The 6th Global Conference, Storytelling, Illness and Medicine, Budapest, Hungary, March 2016).

17   Soddell, "Sound Experience."

18   Ibid.

institutions, and belief systems that promote avoidance or denigration of this journey are dangerous" too, as such journeys are both heroic and necessary.[19]

Collaborative relationships were noted as being of paramount importance when working alongside patients as co-researchers. The health professionals in the group explained how much they had in common with their patients,[20] particularly the importance of being sensitive to their roles as co-authors in the co-construction of their patients' new stories, the language that they shared to do this, and their exploration of what works and what does not.[21] Similarly, in a discussion on patients' use of social media, one presenter suggested that mental health issues like depression are more likely to elicit an appropriate care response if they are "communicated in a culturally recognisable way by the distressed."[22]

However, caution was expressed over assuming that the patient is ignorant of his or her illness and has little to contribute to its understanding, or that the expert professional should always feel the need to provide answers, diagnoses, or ways to ameliorate it.

C   *Inclusivity versus Othering*
        ... elimination of the divide between the able-other and the dis-
        abled self.[23]

It was agreed that medical processes can marginalise and disempower patients, and many of the presentations were designed to show how this situation might be improved by taking relationally supportive positions that accommodate the realities of differently-functioned individuals where understanding, rather than a cure, might be all that's required. Patients are more than the sum of their disabling experiences, and as illness transforms an individual into a

19   Alexandra Fidyk, "Coming Home – A Journey to the Underworld," (paper presented at The 6th Global Conference, Storytelling, Illness and Medicine, Budapest, Hungary, March 2016).

20   Peter Bray " 'One Eye Watching Our Backs': Therapists Share Personal Stories about Practice," (paper presented at The 6th Global Conference, Storytelling, Illness and Medicine, Budapest, Hungary, March 2016).

21   Mirjam Stuij, Agnes Elling, Tineke Abma, " 'starting all over again'. Living with Diabetes and the Quest for Restitution," (paper presented at The 6th Global Conference, Storytelling, Illness and Medicine, Budapest, Hungary, March 2016).

22   Hans Sternudd, "Having the Voice of Depression – An Example of Pathographic Film Narratives on YouTube," (paper presented at The 6th Global Conference, Storytelling, Illness and Medicine, Budapest, Hungary, March 2016).

23   Singh, "Life-writing and the Disabled Self."

patient it can also make them appear to be less than normal or even a bad person.[24]

A commonly held myth about illness is contagion, which assumes that sick people should be kept away from healthy people.[25] "Patients may be tormented with the agonising feelings of being unwanted, helpless with the loss of self-mastery, and deeply-depressed."[26] Similarly, physically disabled individuals may regard themselves as useless because the narrative of the dominant culture reinforces it.[27]

It was noted that whilst medical training often provides information concerning the psychology of the healthy person, it rarely discusses the psychology of those that are unwell.[28] Literature has a significant role here to enable a rapprochement between the able-bodied self and the experiences of the other. Here the work of Oliver Sacks was given as a particular example, "By narrativising the case studies of his patients, he does not merely look at them as objects of medical study but also as subjects of an alternate experience."[29] In addition, it was suggested that schizophrenics are more likely to feel alienated, stigmatised and othered by society because they carry the distorting label of the mentally ill and suffer the consequences of negative stereotyping that prevents their being seen objectively.[30] It was also argued that human beings may not possess the empathic understanding to truly enter and understand another's subjective world. Here anti-stigma practices, that raise awareness through education, can directly challenge false beliefs about mental illness and reveal the humanity of both the patient and their professional helpers. Disclosing identity transformation over time was also a feature of a piece about aging. It explained that because the normative impairments and losses of older populations tend to be gradual in their process and are seen as inevitable they

24 Ana Maria Borlescu, "One Story among Many: Narrative Episodes and the Construction of Doctors' Identities," (paper presented at The 6th Global Conference, Storytelling, Illness and Medicine, Budapest, Hungary, March 2016).
25 Carnelli, "Back to Eden in the 20th-century Europe."
26 Esther Chow and Irene Ip, "Voices of Stroke Survivors in Reconstructing their Preferred Identities: Therapeutic use of Personal Narratives," (paper presented at The 6th Global Conference, Storytelling, Illness and Medicine, Budapest, Hungary, March 2016).
27 Yomna Saber, "Disability in Toni Cade Bambara's *The Salt Eaters*: Narrating Pain and Healing Wound," (paper presented at The 6th Global Conference, Storytelling, Illness and Medicine, Budapest, Hungary, March 2016).
28 Borlescu, "One Story among Many."
29 Singh, "Life-writing and the Disabled Self."
30 Andrew Molas, "Breaking down Barriers: Applying Lugones' Concept of 'World Travelling' to Reduce Stigma Associated with Schizophrenia," (paper presented at The 6th Global Conference, Storytelling, Illness and Medicine, Budapest, Hungary, March 2016).

can be easily disregarded and lead to the invisiblisation and "othering of the old."[31]

Similarly, the issue of people living with undiagnosable or invisible illnesses like fibromyalgia was also raised.[32] It was noted that, as diagnosis is only the formal identification and introduction to a relationship with the disease, credit should be given to the patient for managing their chronic illness for so long. It was also noted that individuals can be highly challenged by diagnoses. To be told that "you look so well" when you know you are not can alienate the sufferer from those that they live with who don't understand the disease or recognise the presence of chronic pain. In turn these patients can reject their diagnoses, refuse treatment or to engage in self-care, "This situation causes the dynamics of the encounter to become entirely different from consultations held with other patients."[33] In short, the conference was challenged to see beyond physical appearances and to understand how patients live with their symptoms – suggesting that society defines pain by its visibility and allocates its compassion and treatment accordingly.

As it was agreed that a patient's visibility may so easily lead to invisibility and then to silence, social engagement with others was regarded as a fundamental aspect of support. Group interventions provide essential opportunities for patient sharing, and the modification of illness narratives that incorporate self-acceptance, understanding and connection. "In therapy, the patient should be assisted to see that he has influence over his illness, transforming him from being managed by the problem to being its manager."[34] It was also suggested that helpers and researchers recognise that illness, although it exists in time, is also made visible in physical spaces and that the unique ways that individuals use and positively benefit from one space, rather than another, be more positively identified.[35]

31   Rasha Salah Fawzy, "Taming Age: the Inevitable Illness," (paper presented at The 6th Global Conference, Storytelling, Illness and Medicine, Budapest, Hungary, March 2016).

32   Tirsa Colmenares and Ingris Peláez-Ballestas "Narratives of an Invisible Social Suffering: Experiences of People with Fibromyalgia," (paper presented at The 6th Global Conference, Storytelling, Illness and Medicine, Budapest, Hungary, March 2016).

33   Ibid.

34   Liat Mor and Yael Efrati "Group Intervention for Women Suffering From Endometriosis, Held at the Center for Treatment of Endometriosis, Sheba Medical Center," (paper presented at The 6th Global Conference, Storytelling, Illness and Medicine, Budapest, Hungary, March 2016).

35   Joan Francisco Matamoros-Sanin, "Spatial Notions and Illness," (paper presented at The 6th Global Conference, Storytelling, Illness and Medicine, Budapest, Hungary, March 2016).

D   *Reclaiming Identity*

Too tired to respond, she briefly relaxes into the role, relinquishing the feminist claim to autonomy and self-determination over her own body.[36]

Illness is feared at a fundamental level because it forces unwanted change and can transform and circumscribe a person's previous identity.[37]

When re-membering personal losses, patients carefully hold a story of their pathway into and out of health but they are necessarily limited by expression and the receptivity of the listener. Most commonly patient narratives include a strong need for restitution – to return to a previous state of health.[38] Sample responses from stroke patients suggest that by accepting manifold losses and gaining a sense of purpose and commitment, mastery and satisfaction, and the cultivation of hope and a positive focus for improvement during the course of recovery, patients can still cherish and utilise what remains to them. Chow and Ip suggest that the will to live in survivors of chronic illness is strong as they are forced to establish new identities that incorporate both their losses and gains. This transition is difficult and its precarious negotiation involves social support and the maintenance of hope.[39]

In terms of patient choice and agency, the conferences challenged itself to understand the patient's reality and to understand how patients and helpers collaboratively and sympathetically negotiate this discrete "space between"?[40] Not surprisingly it was accepted that creative approaches that arise collaboratively from a greater empathic understanding of how the patient uniquely functions in the world, rather than manualised interventions, are preferred by patients and their agency is of paramount concern in these processes.

By speaking out and writing down experiences of illness, patients have more control over how the story is told as it shifts and transforms itself in the telling. It was agreed that a willingness to tell these stories and a place in which to tell them doesn't just happen, people need an invitation to be heard and understood. "Feelings of being valued and the positive impact of being listened to at a time of great personal distress," are what patients require.[41] Thus, it seemed

---

36   Fernández-Morales, "In Me and Everywhere."
37   Naomi Krüger, "Assembling a 'new humanity in the loss': The Problems and Possibilities of Telling Stories about Dementia," (paper presented at The 6th Global Conference, Storytelling, Illness and Medicine, Budapest, Hungary, March 2016).
38   Stuij, Elling, and Abma, "Starting all over again."
39   Chow and Ip, "Voices of Stroke Survivors in Reconstructing their Preferred Identities."
40   Bray "One Eye Watching Our Backs."
41   Youell, Ward and Quinney, "Sharing Stories for Wellbeing."

important that health professionals be encouraged to relinquish some of their expert power and trained to attend to the voices of those that they care for,[42] to embrace the patient and the carer's suffering without fear and with a full heart.[43] The onus is placed upon the listener to attend more closely to the nuances of what is said and left unsaid, and the teller becomes less objectified.[44]

Although attending to patients' versions of their histories requires a sophisticated form of listening and caring, it was suggested that it can also lead to job enhancement for the carer and satisfied patients. "Like the narrative, medical practice requires the engagement of one person with another one and realizes that authentic engagement is transformative for all participants."[45]

> The telling of personal reminiscences was reported to bring positive reminders of changing times and lived experiences. Workshop engagement led some participants to experience improved confidence and reduced social isolation, evidenced through staff and family views and participation in new activities.'[46] In another study it was proposed that use of story-telling in group healing practices, previously disregarded in working with sexual violence trauma, is both a valid and "effective alternative support intervention."[47]

Furthermore, it was suggested that telling stories makes sense of ill-health, especially those narrative that are sustainable and durable. Essentially, patients benefit from sharing stories of illness in a safe and carefully facilitated environment. They recognise that they are not alone and can learn about themselves and their condition from others' feedback and experiences. In an evaluative study of storytelling sessions with individuals in palliative care participants reported autonomy, enjoyment and control when deciding what stories to share.

---

42   Pais, "From Normative to Deviant Behaviour."

43   Deborah Freedman, "AIDS Awakens Ancient Stories," (paper presented at The 6th Global Conference: Storytelling, Illness and Medicine, Budapest, Hungary, March 2016).

44   Victorria Simpson-Gervin, "Narrative Medicine and Storytelling: An Alternative Method for Healing," (paper presented at The 6th Global Conference, Storytelling, Illness and Medicine, Budapest, Hungary, March 2016).

45   Lavinia Bianchi, Susanna Coangelo, Alberto Quagliata, and Mario Cusmai, "I-Learning, Digital Storytelling and Health Care," (paper presented at The 6th Global Conference, Storytelling, Illness and Medicine, Budapest, Hungary, March 2016).

46   Youell, Ward and Quinney, "Sharing Stories for Wellbeing."

47   Elena Sharratt, " 'Group Narratives of Trauma and Healing': Community Storytelling as a Critique of Isolated 'Talk Therapy' amongst Survivors of Sexual Violence," (paper presented at The 6th Global Conference: Storytelling, Illness and Medicine, Budapest, Hungary, March 2016).

Sessions provided an opportunity to make sense of their experiences and "to explore their sense of self and feel valued as a person not a patient."[48]

These stories are very active accounts of patients' conditions, they embody all of their hopes and concerns regarding not only their treatment but how they are and want to be in their lives.[49] To create a new story that makes sense of their experiences of illness they may well incorporate new elements that have to do with managing personal losses, living a good life and taking responsibility for their own health that make this alternative pathway more bearable. It is an exercise in "narrative development and narrative autonomy, i.e. the capacity to bring your actions in line with your sense of self and life story."[50] Although they are still largely untested and may not be suitable for all patients, diary writing and journaling preserve hope, assist in modifying narratives and maintain crucial human connections and relationships. "The diaries weave the different stages of illness and the players (clinician, patient, family) into parallel plots."[51]

Connection and the development of friendships in long-term care seems critical to sustaining self-respect and quality of life, which in turn supports recovery. In a presentation about patient experiences of asylums it was observed that the "emotional connections rather than the physical environment in which the patients stayed"[52] figured most favourably in their narratives.

Finally, it was suggested that accounts of patient experiences in novels and poetry might assist health practitioners to extend their understanding of what it is like to be a patient and to be human. Eve Ensler's memoir was used as an example. Describing her struggle with "her vulnerable self as a patient in a hyper-technological, for-profit health system"[53] it explains how she learned to be a patient with cancer.

Medicine may not have the cure for everything and, it was suggested, that although a diagnosis might go some way to responding to a patient's problem story and even provide a solution, the solution or treatment cannot always lead to a happy ending.

---

48 Youell, Ward and Quinney, "Sharing Stories for Wellbeing."
49 Simpson-Gervin, "Narrative Medicine and Storytelling."
50 Stuij, Elling, and Abma, "Starting all over again."
51 Nihada Besic, Svatka Micik and Krish Sundararajan "You've Never Lost a Fight Even with Dad so you won't Lose this One: Narrative of Critical Illness and Patient Diaries in an Intensive Care Unit," (paper presented at The 6th Global Conference, Storytelling, Illness and Medicine, Budapest, Hungary, March 2016).
52 Calabria, "Insider Stories from the Asylum."
53 Fernández-Morales, "In Me and Everywhere."

5   Afterword

Conference participants from 20 countries confirmed that storytelling, in the context of ill-health and medicine, can generate a wide range of perspectives and discussions. All four themes confirm the importance of interpersonal relationship in healing and it was interesting to see that "non-medical" influences were regarded as either equal to or more important than purely medical interventions. Critically, therefore, the most fundamental question was, "What qualities do patients appreciate and derive benefit from in the professional helpers and organisations that care for them?"

This conference was an opportunity to share stories of heroic, determined, and sometimes difficult patients and simply to present ideas about what human beings say they need when they are sick and what seems to work for those who find themselves in places of care and caring. Consequently, in this analysis "the patient" appears in many guises as a consumer of health, a person of significant research interest, the object of study who is acted upon, and as an agent of their own change. Unsurprisingly, at this conference the patients were not largely the tellers of their own stories but presented as significant characters whose illnesses, diagnoses and experiences and outcomes of subsequent interventions had become irreversibly stitched into their identities. Caught between what they once were and what they were becoming these moving presentations introduced exceptional people, some travelling alone and invisible to society. All on difficult journeys, they just needed help to keep going. Many times that help was warmly shared in deliberately organised collaborations that gave groups and individuals the hope and assistance necessary to return them to a baseline of healthy living, or a place where illness or disability became more manageable.

Bibliography

Besic, Nihada, Svatka Micik and Krish Sundararajan. "You've Never Lost a Fight Even with Dad so you won't Lose this One: Narrative of Critical Illness and Patient Diaries in an Intensive Care Unit." Paper presented at The 6th Global Conference: Storytelling, Illness and Medicine. Budapest, Hungary, March 2016.

Bianchi, Lavinia, Susanna Coangelo, Alberto Quagliata, and Mario Cusmai. "I-Learning, Digital Storytelling and Health Care." Paper presented at The 6th Global Conference: Storytelling, Illness and Medicine. Budapest, Hungary, March 14–16 2016.

Borlescu, Ana Maria. "One Story among Many: Narrative Episodes and the Construction of Doctors' Identities." Paper presented at The 6th Global Conference: Storytelling, Illness and Medicine. Budapest, Hungary, March 14–16 2016.

Braun, Virginia and Victoria Clarke, "Using Thematic Analysis in Psychology." *Qualitative Research in Psychology* (2006): 77–101.

Bray, Peter. " 'One Eye Watching Our Backs': Therapists Share Personal Stories about Practice." Paper presented at The 6th Global Conference: Storytelling, Illness and Medicine. Budapest, Hungary, March 14–16 2016.

Bray, Peter and Ana Borlescu, eds. *Beyond Present Patient Realities: Collaboration, Care and Identity.* Oxford, England: Inter-Disciplinary Press, 2015.

Calabria, Verusca. "Insider Stories from the Asylum: Exploring Peer and Staff-Patient Relationships." Paper presented at The 6th Global Conference: Storytelling, Illness and Medicine. Budapest, Hungary, March 14-16 2016.

Carnelli, Silvia, "Back to Eden in the 20th-century Europe: Monte Verità & Glastonbury. (Hi)Stories from two 'alternative' Isles of Healing.' " Paper presented at The 6th Global Conference: Storytelling, Illness and Medicine. Budapest, Hungary, March 14–16 2016.

Chow, Esther and Irene Ip. "Voices of Stroke Survivors in Reconstructing their Preferred Identities: Therapeutic use of Personal Narratives." Paper presented at The 6th Global Conference: Storytelling, Illness and Medicine. Budapest, Hungary, March 14–16 2016.

Colmenares, Tirsa and Ingris Peláez-Ballestas. "Narratives of an Invisible Social Suffering: Experiences of People with Fibromyalgia." Paper presented at The 6th Global Conference: Storytelling, Illness and Medicine. Budapest, Hungary, March 14–16 2016.

Fawzy, Rasha Salah. "Taming Age: the Inevitable Illness." Paper presented at The 6th Global Conference: Storytelling, Illness and Medicine. Budapest, Hungary, March 14–16 2016.

Fernández-Morales, Marta. "In Me and Everywhere: Making Meaning of Cancer' citing Eve Ensler in Eve Ensler's memoir *In the Body of the World.*" Paper presented at The 6th Global Conference: Storytelling, Illness and Medicine. Budapest, Hungary, March 14-16 2016.

Fidyk, Alexandra. "Coming Home – A Journey to the Underworld." Paper presented at The 6th Global Conference: Storytelling, Illness and Medicine. Budapest, Hungary, March 14–16 2016.

Freedman, Deborah. "AIDS Awakens Ancient Stories." Paper presented at The 6th Global Conference: Storytelling, Illness and Medicine. Budapest, Hungary, March 14–16 2016.

Jajszczok, Justyna. "The Stories of Invading Microbes: Infection Literature." Paper presented at The 6th Global Conference: Storytelling, Illness and Medicine. Budapest, Hungary, March 14–16 2016.

Krüger, Naomi. "Assembling a 'new humanity in the loss': The Problems and Possibilities of Telling Stories about Dementia." Paper presented at The 6th Global Conference: Storytelling, Illness and Medicine. Budapest, Hungary, March 14–16 2016.

Matamoros-Sanin, Joan Francisco. "Spatial Notions and Illness." Paper presented at The 6th Global Conference: Storytelling, Illness and Medicine. Budapest, Hungary, March 14–16 2016.

Molas, Andrew. "Breaking down Barriers: Applying Lugones' Concept of 'World Travelling' to Reduce Stigma Associated with Schizophrenia." Paper presented at The 6th Global Conference: Storytelling, Illness and Medicine. Budapest, Hungary, March 14–16 2016.

Mor, Liat and Yael Efrati. "Group Intervention for Women Suffering From Endometriosis, Held at the Center for Treatment of Endometriosis, Sheba Medical Center." Paper presented at The 6th Global Conference: Storytelling, Illness and Medicine. Budapest, Hungary, March 14–16 2016.

Pais, Sofia Castanheira. "From Normative to Deviant Behaviour: Health and Illness Definitions Related to Children and Adolescents' Perspectives." Paper presented at The 6th Global Conference: Storytelling, Illness and Medicine. Budapest, Hungary, March 14–16 2016.

Saber, Yomna. "Disability in Toni Cade Bambara's *The Salt Eaters*: Narrating Pain and Healing Wound." Paper presented at The 6th Global Conference: Storytelling, Illness and Medicine. Budapest, Hungary, March 14–16 2016.

Sharratt, Elena. " 'Group Narratives of Trauma and Healing': Community Storytelling as a Critique of Isolated 'Talk Therapy' amongst Survivors of Sexual Violence." Paper presented at The 6th Global Conference: Storytelling, Illness and Medicine. Budapest, Hungary, March 14–16 2016.

Simpson-Gervin, Victorria. "Narrative Medicine and Storytelling: An Alternative Method for Healing." Paper presented at The 6th Global Conference: Storytelling, Illness and Medicine. Budapest, Hungary, March 14–16 2016.

Singh, Sandeep. "Life-writing and the Disabled Self: Discourses on Subjectivity." Paper presented at The 6th Global Conference: Storytelling, Illness and Medicine. Budapest, Hungary, March 14–16 2016.

Soddell, Thembi. "Sound Experience: Listening Session and Discussion on the Experience of Invisible Illness." Paper presented at The 6th Global Conference: Storytelling, Illness and Medicine. Budapest, Hungary, March 14–16 2016.

Sternudd, Hans. "Having the Voice of Depression – An Example of Pathographic Film Narratives on YouTube." Paper presented at The 6th Global Conference: Storytelling, Illness and Medicine. Budapest, Hungary, March 14–16 2016.

Stuij , Mirjam, Agnes Elling, Tineke Abma. " 'Starting all over again'. Living with Diabetes and the Quest for Restitution." Paper presented at The 6th Global Conference: Storytelling, Illness and Medicine. Budapest, Hungary, March 14–16 2016.

Youell, Jane, Alison Ward and Miranda Quinney. "Sharing Stories for Wellbeing." Paper presented at The 6th Global Conference: Storytelling, Illness and Medicine. Budapest, Hungary, March 14–16 2016.

CHAPTER 7

Beginning to Breathe

Peter Bray

1 Introduction

In June, 2010, I was presenting a paper at an international transpersonal psychology conference in Moscow. As part of the experience I had elected to attend a two-day Holotropic Breathwork workshop led by Stanislav Grof one of the founders of transpersonal psychology.[1]

As a scholar of Grof I had some idea of what the experience might be like but was troubled by my father's imminent death.[2]

2 A Case Study

Day 1 - Beginning.[a]	Day 2 - Breathing.[j]
Introducing the Experience.	Anticipation.
The monotheistic materialism of industrial society pathologises spirituality...	In a Moscow hotel conference room with 80 strangers. Scattered haphazardly across the floor perched on mats, chattering a rainbow
Hindu experiential, spiritual exercises, like yoga, raise awareness and explore the energy that is identical to that found in the universe.	of languages to colleagues and new friends. There are people everywhere rearranging blankets and personal belongings to take full advantage of newly claimed spaces. I carefully pick my way through the excited

---

1 Miles A. Vich, 'Some Historical Sources of the Term "Transpersonal"', *Journal of Transpersonal Psychology* 20 (1988): 107–110, notes that Abraham Maslow began using the word 'transpersonal' – meaning 'across or beyond the individual person or psyche' – in his correspondence with Stanislav Grof, transpersonal psychology's co-founder, in the mid 1960's.

2 Over the last half century Stanslav Grof has written a number of books that have outlined his cartography of the psyche such as *Beyond the Brain: Birth, Death and Transcendence in Psychotherapy* (Albany: State University New York Press, 1985), and *The Holotropic Mind: The Three Levels of Human Consciousness and How They Shape Our* Lives (New York: Harper Collins, 1993). However, *Holotropic Breathwork: A New Approach to Self-Exploration and Therapy* (New York: SUNY, 2010), written with Christina Grof, provides a rationale and a description of the intervention in practice.

Ultimately we are all identical with that identity...Moving from body ego identification to identification with the source...sometimes small steps...sometimes breakthroughs.

bodies towards my Belgian sitter who worked with me yesterday and ready myself to experience the deep breathing and evocative music that will allow me to explore the deeper dynamics of my psyche.

These experiences have a quality of numinosity... They are the software of the psyche. Working with holotropic states it is virtually impossible to use the intellect to understand the psyche.

Sitters...
Don't leave the breather.

Preparation.
I begin by discarding items of clothing that can obstruct the therapeutic process such as shoes, jewellery, glasses and connections to cyberspace. Thus, as an unencumbered breather I lie on my back on a thin mattress with my head resting on a small pillow.

From a strictly materialistic point of view, if you have spiritual experiences...there is something wrong with you. You are not educated and you get a diagnosis.
...In Brahma the questions asked are 'Who are you? Who am I?'
The answer given is,

My sitter, a complete stranger until today, positions himself comfortably next to me preparing for the three hours observation that will ensue. With a box of tissues and a bottle of water close to hand, he has clear instructions not to leave me on my own.

'You are god. You are divine.'

'What do they think I am going to do....?'

'...A divine spark!'

Whilst waiting, we loudly amuse ourselves with possible fantasy scenarios.

Cynicism.
The day before I had been Carl's sitter and had been impressed by his gymnastic convulsions as the breather. Later, I was more than put out when he cryptically suggested that,
'Nothing happened.'

Even to different therapies, there is a challenge in understanding the potential of 'altered states' of consciousness.
Each will tell you something different about what is wrong with you, and how you should do your therapy.

This didn't help at all.
I wasn't about to be satisfied with anything other than a fully aware, deeply penetrative and significant plunge into the inner workings of my complex psyche. I hadn't travelled half way around the globe, overcoming all sorts of personal and professional demons, to claim anything less!

Respect your own uniquely individual authority.
Holotropic Breathwork uses the power of the
inner healer.

The facilitator will focus the breathers on their
bodies so that they become aware of aches and
pains as they begin to practice and focus on
mindful relaxation.

Working with connected/circular breathing that
is a little faster than usual...work out what suits
your personal style.

...To aid the process of relaxation I want you to
visualise a light passing slowly over your body,
scanning and soothing it as it moves upwards
from your toes to your head.

Experience the deep comfort of having someone
there.
As the rhythmic music...is played quite loudly the
breather is encouraged to deepen and speed up
their breathing above normal.
...mindful...
relaxation...

You as the healer are kept in control - use the
word 'stop' to get the attention and support from
your sitter or trained facilitators to stop whatever
they are doing for you. Any other words might
be part of the healing process...part of the inner
dialogue.

Body Awareness.
On my back with my eyes closed, arms
resting by my sides, palms turned up to
accept the experience, I feel a level of
unaccustomed anxiety and vulnerability.

I am ready to begin but my mind is making
excuses to leave the room.

Support.
Now, the slow heavy voice of the facilitator
breaks my reverie forcing me to connect to
reality and to the exercise...

Supine, each wave of gently directed probing
sends me deeper into a warmer and more
accepting state.

Breathing.
In this place of soft consciousness I am
fully aware: sensing others around me; the
air conditioning; incidental noises in the
building; and random thoughts that become
easier and easier to resist and then put away.

Instead of feeling uncomfortable about
maintaining a slightly heavier and faster
breathing routine the rhythmic rising and
falling of my chest feels reassuring and
natural. Simultaneously, the strong and
evocative beat of aboriginal music fills the
room and I am aware that my muscles are
responding to the changes in my breathing.

Trust.
My eyes are closed in a room with 80
strangers. Yet, I am giving my body over
to its own intelligence and it feels right.
In the emerging inner peace I feel myself
trusting my sitter and the process. I am
being comfortably held by other forces - the
paradoxical tension between holding on to
self control and letting go.

I feel ready for anything!

Individuals may experience the trauma of abuse or experiences of not receiving, or being denied something.
The breather has a right to refuse assistance.

What might my body do that it hasn't done before and where might my mind rove?

I am a white middle aged, middle class male...surprise me!

Everything is created by consciousness; there is nothing that cannot be experienced. It can do things that the brain by itself cannot possibly do.

Music.
Soon the flowing music becomes the only way to judge the passing of time. I am floating just below its surface, observing with some relish and without the need to interpret or interfere that my body, or rather the muscles, are gently rippling to their own rhythms and cadences.

Like radar...the holotropic state finds the areas in the unconscious which are most relevant - that have the strongest emotional charge. That will be the part that surfaces into consciousness.

My body is doing what it wants and I feel an unaccustomed sense of surrender.

As the body ego dissolves we can subjectively share in the experiences of all life forms...a very wide spectrum of experience

With an unfolding calm in my centre and a growing trust in the process, I am able to luxuriate in the warmth of just being.

The collective unconscious incorporates a record of human history...Anima mundi!

The music is deeply rhythmical like the beat of a heart, my heart. I revel in its spaciousness.

A whole record or history of experience is accessible from the Basic Perinatal Matrices.[b]

I am at once a container, a vehicle, a stage, a canvas of universal human expression and connection. United with this flowing cosmic landscape an ancient pulse begs my body to respond.

Relived through large archetypal experiences and images in the transpersonal realm of experience...

Momentarily my detached and reluctant intellect breaks loose toward the surface.

...Is this too soon, and how is this to work?

Our individual psyche contains the whole universe.[c]
The psyche is the ultimate mystery. There is no way to figure it out with the intellect.
In holotropic states we can get over boundaries, we can transcend them. But there needs to be a safe context. Sitters, see to it that the breather doesn't move too far. Use soft materials to restrain him. To prevent injury or physical impact that influences the breather's or other breathers' experiences.

In unquestionable response my arm gently detaches itself from the mat and rises snake-like, charming my mind into silence. The intelligence that guides my arm permits the other parts of my body to meet their own desires and resolve their own issues.

The breathing causes spasms...the music induces deep tensions associated with traumatic experiences...Physical contact can be offered that will enable and unblock these experiences and help the individual understand what they mean. 'By experiencing them, people are getting rid of them.'[xl]

Inner Intelligence.
Without seeing I feel inner healing unfolding with certainty, grace and purposeful eloquence. I am opening and it is liberating as my limbs wrap around each other and dance.

It seems counter-intuitive...rather than controlling them, the breather is asked to attend to these physical tensions...even to vocalise.

My torso pulses and my legs work expansively, my arms twist and flex, swooping and gliding while it falls to my hands to articulate the subtleties of deep unexpressed emotion. I am being comfortably held by my own body, aware of its indecipherable choreography and marvelling at its effortless movements.

Different psychosomatic disorders can present themselves in the body. This is where the bodywork is useful.

Earlier we had been asked to anchor our thoughts upon some particular source of strength. I had tried to focus on God but couldn't sustain it.

One major observation or one category of experience, from thanatology, is that in certain near-death situations consciousness leaves the body.

At this moment, on this day, in my first breath work session I couldn't avoid the fact, nor remove it from my mind, that my father of 89 years was dying in a cottage-hospital bed in Norfolk, England. The unavoidable realisation held me hostage. Dad is dying and I am in Moscow.
'There is nothing you can do for him now. We just have to wait.'

Reconciliation.
On a mat on a Moscow floor. Here is Dad.

Our individual psyche is a microcosm that contains the whole universe...

If you work with the holotropic model of the psyche the roots go to deep levels.

I can see him so vividly in the early English morning. His head is buttressed by painfully large pillows. The sun patterns the bed clothes and outlines his awkward frailty caged in that vast metal bed. He has become a fraction of a man, an angular frame of translucently pale skin on bone. His chest slowly and painfully rises and falls as he fights for each rasping breath. His mouth, now permanently open, receives only extra oxygen as tubes feed and lead away to boxy machines on stands.

'If we have emotional problems, psychosomatic problems, or problems in relation to other people, the roots are not just in our biography but there are also additional roots connected to the trauma of birth...and even, what we call the transpersonal level.'[e]

I am engulfed by a wave of uncontrollable sadness, a dark void of extraordinary loss. My body responding to these new emotions gulps and drowns in their depths. My orientation is confused...
am I descending or ascending? Is it my experience or my father's?

Relax enough to enjoy the present and leave the intellect behind.

In spite of my total absorption I am aware of the others working through their processes. They sigh and shout, make vomiting noises and cry in strange accompaniment to the seemingly permanent backdrop of evocative music.

To overcome these problems you need to work through the different levels. It must be experiential. The bad news is that there are many levels to manage.

Even as I am inexorably drawn back into my journey I join them. My vocalisations are timid at first but turn by degrees into a robust appreciation and identification with emotions of loss. I am an outpouring of wailing and tears in a womb of comfortingly soft translucent shapes. Now, suddenly propelled through these emotionally drenched forms I struggle with buffeting changes of pressure.

Tensions will build up and then there will be some relaxation...

Union.
I feel warmth and then tension in my arms. Unseen hands have gripped them and are firmly pulling them upwards. For the

Certain assisted body work may also be required for individuals who experience a block that needs to be worked out; otherwise individuals allow their bodies to express their needs at that time while under the supervision of a caring sitter.

first time I am aware of another physical presence, an actual intelligence, and in that moment I understand. I am allowed to fully own these desperate feelings of sadness and longing and yet powerfully I identify my father's presence. How can I sufficiently describe the completeness of our delicate entwinement? My feelings are his feelings. I am experiencing his pain, his shortness of breath. I am his anger at having to leave a life unfinished, a rude severing from family and dreams.

In this hermetic vessel, and through the exchange of symbolic language, the intellect converses with the transpersonal and transformation can take place.[f]

Fused with him I understand that I am so much more, that there is so much more. Our hunger for life and pleasure in what we are sets us spinning in a climactic vortex and in

this final movement we are the music and
the players; we are their instruments and
scores, the concert hall and the audience.
Feeling what he feels and thinking his
thoughts we glimpse a 'heaven' Dad claimed
not to believe in.
Death or life beyond still summons and tugs
with cruel insistence.
'We are so tired Dad'.
'How are you holding on Dad?'
I can quite clearly see my mother and my
aunt sitting by the bed helplessly witnessing
and intuitively understanding Dad's
unrelenting struggle. I can feel it and it fills
me with dread. His life and his loss are ours
and it hurts. Caught between the certainty of
life and the uncertainty of death I linger with
my Dad in that place that is more womb
than world and feel his fear and his inertia
as my own.
I try to comfort him with my presence and
a trickle of warmth comes back in response.
I feel recognised, almost understood.
Unexpectedly, this understanding is
interrupted by another. A firm but
kindly voice that I don't recognise at all
addresses us.
'It will be alright', it says.
'Let go now. It's okay to just let go.'

Understanding.
I feel Dad relax but he is so tightly bound
to the earth that he finds it hard to move;
the bed, the blankets, the air line, the
drip, the familiar voices all serve to bind
him to the present. Then it seems that my
outstretched arms find new purpose. Still
raised, my hands seek the body of my father
but I am myself again and recognise my
extraordinary loss. I ache to hug him but
I know I can't allow myself to prolong his
pain by physically tying him to me. As if in
acknowledgement I feel his warmth again.
Tears are streaming down my face.
'So many losses, so many to lose', comes the
voice but this time it is all directed at me.
I feel wracked with the grief of all humanity
and it is bitter sweet.

Gift.

I feel wave upon wave of tension release itself as I give up my father to his bliss and my tears of pain turn to tears of great joy. My hands, still wishing to claim what was lost, come together as if to receive or shape something and a globe of soft light appears above me and gently floats down into them. I am surprised and at the same time receive it unquestioningly. I understand it to be something of my father that has been tenderly and lovingly formed and is at that moment being channelled into my waiting hands. Of their own volition they mirror the sphere and guide it downward as it pushes itself into my chest. I watch all this with a degree of detachment not altogether understanding its significance. It is what it is. However, as the process concludes a huge smile immediately suffuses my face and I quite literally light up with relief and joy. Dad and I have been together – we are together! We shared an extraordinary moment and he has given me something, something wonderful and inexplicable, a great treasure. It seems to me now that he is free in a way that I can only just conceive and I know with absolute certainty that he is alright – that we are alright!

*'A typical result...is profound emotional release and physical relaxation...people report that they feel more relaxed than they have ever felt in their life. Continued accelerated breathing thus represents an extremely powerful and effective method of stress reduction and it is conducive to emotional and psychosomatic healing. Another frequent result of this work is connection with the numinous dimensions of one's own psyche and of existence in general.'*⁸

Dazzled.

I open my eyes in a room full of unique and precious individuals.

It is as if I have entered that room for the first time. I suddenly become aware that there are people everywhere: facilitators and sitters purposefully tend to their breathers; breathers busily work with inner processes or come in to land; and the room thrums with their energy and light. I am dazzled by the brightness and colour of the unfolding scene and the forgotten impact of the music. Momentarily my senses reel as I try to take it in, and all the time the broad grin doesn't leave my face and the warm glow suffuses my whole being.

'Are you okay?'

After a while a facilitator comes over and hunkers down...

...When you feel you have landed then go and draw a mandala and share your experiences in a group.[h]	I can't wipe the smile from my face as I reply, 'I have never felt better'. And I mean it.
'In the terminal stage of the session...Intimate contact with nature can also have a very calming and grounding effect and help the integration of the session.'[i]	Carl carefully assists me from the room. I have been 'breathing' for over two hours but have no notion of the time. It is only later that I look at my phone and see that my sister in England has sent me a text message. It reads quite simply,
I went outside and into the park...	'Sorry. Dad has left us - big hug xxx'

a   Unless additionally referenced, the italicised text in this column is taken from notes made at Stanislav Grof's morning lecture, preparatory to author's holotropic breathwork session on Monday, 21st June, 2010.

b   Stan Grof conceives of four Basic Perinatal Matrices, corresponding to the four consecutive periods of biological delivery, which make up a unique and fundamental biological and existential perinatal dimension that bridges biographical and transpersonal experiences enabling a level of universal consciousness ordinarily beyond the individual's reach. Source, Stanislav Grof, *The Holotropic Mind* (New York: Harper Collins, 1993).

c   Richard Tarnas, *Cosmos and Psyche: Intimations of a New World View*, (New York: Viking, 2006).

d   "Christina and Stan Grof: Holotropic Breathwork", viewed December 5, 2017, http://www.youtube.com/watch?feature=player_embedded&v=YVILRQ4gHBk

e   Ibid.

f   See Carl Gustav Jung on the individuation process in Claire and Richard Winston, trans., Aniele Jaffe, ed., *Memories, Dreams, Reflections*, (New York: Random House, Inc. 1989): 209.

g   Stanislav Grof, "Holotropic Breathwork: New Perspectives in Psychotherapy and Self-Exploration," https://www.wisdomuniversity.org/grof/module/week3/pdf/Holotropic%20Breathwork.pdf

h   Drawing mandalas from a meditative state of mind assists participants to externalise, understand, and support themselves, their experiences, and their continuing process.

i   Grof, "Holotropic Breathwork: New Perspectives," 31.

j   Text taken from the author's unpublished experience of a Holotropic Breathwork session entitled, "Beginning to Breathe," written on 23rd June, 2010.

3   Drawing a Mandala

As the events of the session further unfolded and my father's death becomes a reality, I returned to my world disoriented and dreamy. I didn't draw a mandala to help me understand myself or integrate the experience but I did seek the reassuring companionship of fellow participants.

Much later, although unaware of the growth of subtle conscious senses, I was cognisant of the session's solace and its support in the management of the difficult events that surrounded my father's death. A new nurturing spaciousness has been introduced into my day-to-day living and a profound reassurance that I have the capacity as a human being to heal myself. I have developed a more expansive view of personal experience and value the simplicity of attending to breathing and its potential outcomes.

If saying goodbye to dad was only a reassuring delusion ...? It worked for me.

Bibliography

Grof, Stanislav. *Beyond the Brain: Birth, Death and Transcendence in Psychotherapy.* Albany: State University New York Press, 1985.

Grof, Stanislav. *The Holotropic Mind: The Three Levels of Human Consciousness and How They Shape Our Lives.* New York: Harper Collins, 1993.

Grof, Stanislav and Christina Grof. *Holotropic Breathwork: A New Approach to Self-Exploration and Therapy.* New York: SUNY, 2010.

Jung, Carl Gustav, Claire and Richard Winston, trans., Aniele Jaffe, ed. *Memories, Dreams, Reflections.* New York: Random House, Inc. 1989.

Tarnas, Richard. *Cosmos and Psyche: Intimations of a New World View.* New York: Viking, 2006.

Vich, Miles A. 'Some Historical Sources of the Term "Transpersonal." ' *Journal of Transpersonal Psychology*, 20 (1988): 107–110.

CHAPTER 8

Catching Stories: Building a House for Narrative and Communication in Digital Healthcare

Susana Teixeira Magalhães

1   How Fiction Reminds Us of Who We Are

In *The Wounded Storyteller*, Arthur W. Frank defines three types of narratives of illness: restitution stories, that "attempt to outdistance mortality by rendering illness transitory"; chaos stories that "are sucked into the undertow of illness and the disasters that attend it"; and quest stories that "meet suffering head on, they accept illness and seek to use it. Illness is the occasion of a journey that becomes a quest."[1] In order to open a gap that allows possibility to crack out of the nightmare, the storyteller has to go through all of the three types of narrative, much like the characters of Picoult's novel, *The Storyteller*, which was inspired by Simon Wiesenthal, the Nazi-hunter and his book, *The Sunflower*. Wiesenthal writes about his days in a German concentration camp, where he was summoned to the death bed of an SS man who wanted to confess his guilt and be forgiven by a Jew.

In *The Storyteller* there are four parallel stories, embedded narratives like Chinese boxes. Sage is an outstanding baker who works at night and leads a loner existence in a small town. The scar on her face is kept as a secret, pointing out to gloomy past events and precluding her from having a normal life. The shadows of the past seem to push her into painful experiences: the relationship with a funeral director called Adam, who also happens to be married, seems to be a fine arrangement initially, but she ends up suffering as she feels excluded from her lover's life; she is drawn to Josef, a member of the grief group she attends after her mother's death, who confesses to her that he was a Nazi commander in the Holocaust at the Auschwitz concentration camp and asks her to help him die. Minka, Sage's grandmother, grows up in Lodz and is sent to the ghetto with her family. Eventually she is taken to Auschwitz and we closely follow the story of all the hardships she endures and ultimately survives. Franz and Reiner

---

1   Arthur.W. Frank, *The Wounded Storyteller: Body, Illness and Ethics*, 2nd. ed. (Chicago and London: University of Chicago Press, 1995), 115.

are two German brothers who end up in the SS and who play totally different roles due to their different characters: one is serious and sensitive, loyal to his friends and able to praise the fundamental values of life; the other is a callous fighter, obsessed with the duty of acting according to the Nazi ideology. There is another story running alongside Sage's: a wonderful allegory written by Minka, a dark gothic romance about a baker's daughter and two demon brothers who terrorize a village. The novel structure and its plot point respectively to the stories that are always entangled in other stories and to the role of forgiveness and promise in giving a future to the self that comes to be in the story being told.

All the horror of the unbearable suffering in Auschwitz and the void that swallowed the victims of genocide are realities that inhabit a very different territory from that of illness. However, what allows us to draw this parallel between Picoult's novel and narratives of illness is precisely the role of memory in the quest for meaning, for a narrative identity and for the restitution of the possibility of moving on to the future: "[E]vents like the Holocaust and the great crimes of the twentieth century, situated at the limits of representation, stand in the name of all the events that have left their traumatic imprint on hearts and bodies: they protest that they were and as such they demand being said, recounted, understood."[2]

When Josef and Sage meet at a grief group session, they are both living chaotic stories and both are looking for forgiveness and for a different closure or for an exit out of bad memory into the possibility of a future. Bad memory does not let them follow the linear movement of humankind, the same movement that, according to Hannah Arendt in *The Human Condition*, frees us from the cyclical movement of everything else in our world. Sage and Josef are stuck in the past, both carrying the burden of incoherent identity narratives: the former due to the guilt she feels for her mother's death at the car crash while she was driving; the latter, for having been a Nazi commander in the Holocaust at the Auschwitz concentration camp.

The grief group is a place where words count, where narratives are used to search for the good memory, the one that does not enclose oneself into repetitive gestures that prevent oneself from looking into the wound and into the trauma. By sharing with each other their losses, their guilt, their anxiety and need for hope, the members of the group assume their incapacity to forget the lost object, to mourn their loss in order to go on with their lives. Ricoeur states that the critical use of memory is the one that allows us to rise above, freeing

2   Paul Ricoeur, "The Difficulty to Forgive." *Memory, Narrativity, Self and the Challenge to Think God: The Reception within Theology of the Recent Work of Paul Ricoeur*, ed. M. Junker-Kenny and P. Kenny (New York and London: Transactions Publishers, 2004), 498.

oneself from both the excess of memory and the lack of memory, opening up space for promise. Compulsion to repetition and melancholia are the consequences of a blocked memory; the alternative is to remember. Remembrance gives a future to memory. It is important to notice that throughout the novel we are faced with the work of remembering repressed memories by Sage, Josef, Minka, and these entangled stories of remembrance start with Josef's request to be pardoned by Sage—representative of the Jewish people—and to be killed by her as a punishment that would free him from being engulfed in repetition:

> (...) before you help me die, Sage, I need one more favour from you. I ask
>   you to forgive me first.
> "Forgive you?"
> "For the things I did back then."
> "I'm not the one you should be asking for forgiveness for."
> "No," he agrees, "but they are all dead."[3]

Pardon and vengeance are not compatible, because, as Ricoeur states, pardon allows for catharsis to take place and makes a benevolent sacred emerge from it. So, pardon is a kind of gift, originating from the victim and only by pardoning can good oblivion emerge:

> [W]hat kind of forgetting would deserve to be held as a trace of forgiving? I would suggest to speak of a good oblivion in the same way as we speak of a good memory ... Good oblivion should be on the side of this other figure of forgetting, the preservation of the traces, but delivered from their mischievousness, their haunting power. Lifting the burden of the debt is recovering the lightness of existence, the divine freedom from worry.[4]

The uncoupling of the evil from the agent is enacted in the novel with the topos of the Double personified in Reiner and Franz: Reiner assumes his incapacity to feel repentance, and it is instead Franz who repents and asks for forgiveness. However, for Franz there is no future in the request, and what follows is thus the need to have Sage kill him. By not assuming his identity (he claims to be his brother Reiner), Franz cannot be forgiven, because he lacks self-attestation. Remembering is an act where the self recognizes itself. The

---

3 Jodi Picoult, *The Storyteller* (London: Hodder & Stoughton, 2013), 117–118.
4 Paul Ricoeur. *Memory, History, Forgetting.* trans. Kathleen Blamey and David Pellauer (Chicago: University of Chicago Press, 2004), 14–15.

attestation of memories implies an act of self attestation, because attestation is ultimately attestation of the self. Without assuming his own self—*what* and *who he is*—, Franz cannot recognize himself in his memories, and without recognition, there is no forgiveness and hence no future. In spite of his former wisdom—"Don't forget where you came from," he told his brother, trying to make him feel repentance for his violence—, Franz gets stuck in the different possibilities of action that he eagerly looks for in Minka's tale. The story Minka was writing at the concentration camp could have different endings and Franz kept her alive because he wanted to keep the promise of a different future also alive. In a dialogue with his brother Reiner, Franz says that "power isn't doing something terrible to someone who's weaker than you, Reiner. It's having the strength to do something terrible and choosing not to."[5] The capacity to narrate oneself is deeply linked to attestation,[6] ascribing to oneself several actions as one's own or, on the contrary, denying one's involvement in some. To choose one action instead of another is a matter of commitment, an act of freedom and responsibility:

> How does it end? Josef had asked. Now I realize he lied twice to me yesterday: he knew who my grandmother was. Maybe he has hoped I'd lead him to her. Not to kill her (...), but for closure. The monster and the girl who could rescue him: obviously he was reading his life story into her fiction. It was why he had saved her years ago; it was why now he needed to know if he would be redeemed or condemned. And yet the joke was on him, because my grandmother never finished her story. Not because she didn't know the ending; and not because she did (...) and couldn't bear to write it. She had left it blank on purpose, like a postmodern canvas. If you end your story, it's a static work of art, a finite circle. But, if you don't, it belongs to anyone's imagination. It stays alive forever.[7]

---

5 Picoult, *The Storyteller*, 164.
6 See the definition of Self-Attestation by Paul Ricoeur in *Oneself as Another*: 'attestation can be defined as the assurance of being oneself acting and suffering. This assurance remains the ultimate recourse against all suspicion; even if it is always in some sense received from another, it still remains self-attestation. It is self-attestation that at every level—linguistic, praxis, narrative and prescriptive—will preserve the question "who?" from being replaced by questions of "what?" and "why?" Conversely, at the center of the aporia, only the persistence of the question "who?"—in a way laid bare for lack of a response—will reveal itself to be the impregnable refuge for attestation.'
7 Picoult, *The Storyteller*, 527–528.

In the territory of illness, the same search for closure is present. A. W. Frank points out in *The Wounded Storyteller* that illness stories face the task of ordering the chaos of a narrative that was interrupted, while at the same time they must tell the truth about the ongoing interruptions in the future. There is a need of closure and a commitment to the truth of indeterminacy, openness, the awareness that there are no tidy ends. Self-attestation implies facing openness and assuming one's body as the place where the journey of illness develops, as the instrument available to tell one's own narrative, as well as the subject of this narrative. Without self-attestation, there is no memory, no forgiveness, no future.

2   Catching Stories: a Digital House for Reflective Writing and Communication in Health Care

The need to provide all participants in the patient's journey with space for reflective writing practice and for communication has motivated us to create *Catching Stories: A Narrative Medicine Platform*, where patients, caregivers and physicians can write parallel charts[8] and keep up a communication pathway along the illness journey. The challenge we are facing in our digital world is how to enact a narrative approach in healthcare. Is it possible to build a new therapeutic alliance in the digital era? We believe it is, so we have designed the platform *Catching stories* as a pathway for narrative and communication in healthcare. This platform is designed as a house with doors and windows that can be opened (according to ethical and legal norms) by patients, relatives, doctors and other caregivers in order to foster communication and to provide narrative input that can be developed when face-to-face encounter takes place. Health information systems used to be business, professional and organizational-oriented, thus conceiving of the patient as a passive subject and not as an active participant. However, the role of the patient has been changing from passive to active, due to internet-based resources of health information and to a narrative-based approach to the doctor/patient encounter that elicits shared decision making. This approach is firmly rooted in the field of narrative-based medicine, which has been developed by Rita Charon and her Columbia University team since 2000, when the Narrative Medicine Program was implemented at this university. The need to counterbalance evidence-based medicine with

---

8   Rita Charon, *Changing the Face of Medicine*, viewed 29 July 2016, http://www.nlm.nih.gov/changingthefaceofmedicine/video/58_1_trans.html.

relational-based medicine results from the separation that clinical technologies have created between clinicians, caregivers and patients. Bridging the gap between (otherwise) a more impersonal and dehumanizing healthcare environment and the individual illness experience, the focus on the patient's own interpretation of his/her health journey also led to the creation of DIPEX in 2001: Andrew Herxheimer, a clinical pharmacologist, and Ann McPherson, a GP in Oxford, had the original idea of setting up a database of people's accounts of their experience of hospital treatments. The database was intended to complement the Cochrane Library (which reports on the best evidence from medical treatment trials) and help people facing treatment decisions to choose what to do. Our platform of narrative medicine intends to provide patients, physicians and caregivers with the opportunity to register their individual and unique perspective of the health journey they are undertaking, bridging gaps of knowledge and of communication and ensuring narrative inputs for doctor/patients encounters. We assume that the reflective writing practice by each of the participants and the opportunity to decide what they want and are allowed to share with each other has positive impact, leading to:

- higher adherence to therapy and more positive perspective on the health experience (patient);
- less burnout and more solid and effective decision-making resources (caregiver);
- effective shared decision-making tools, more rewarding relationships with patients, caregivers and medical team, and narrative capacities that will eventually contribute to tackle conflicting situations, as those related to medical harm (physician).
- the opportunity to voice their own story, to be listened to attentively, to listen to each other, to take part as active agents in the illness journey (all the participants)

The Storyteller is meaningful in the search for each character's own voice, the voice of the body in relation to the other as a body outside mine, but also as the body that has to do with me and I with it, the so called dyadic body according to A.W. Frank:

> Illness presents a particular opening to becoming a dyadic body, because the ill person is immersed in a suffering that is both wholly individual— my pain is mine alone—but also shared. (...) Storytelling is one medium through which the dyadic body both offers its own pain and receives the reassurance that others recognize what afflicts it.[9]

---

9 Frank, *The Wounded Storyteller*, 36.

The tragedy of not choosing the right way or not choosing any way at all, i.e. choosing not to decide, is present in illness experience and in *The Storyteller*. Sage knows that her relationship with her married lover is wrong, and yet she insists in keeping this affair going; Josef knows from the start that his brother was doing evil, being therefore aware of his own evil as part of the Nazi machine, and yet he does what is expected from him; Leo hunts Nazis for the sake of justice, or is he looking for vengeance? There is no black and white, good and evil, but a lot of gray areas demanding that one chooses between bad and worse. Wisdom is thus portrayed as asking for more (or, in another sense) for less than reason. Narrative allows patients, health professionals and caregivers to share expectations, anxiety, fears and doubts, thus promoting dialogue and shared decision making: "The narrative provides meaning, context, and perspective for the patient's predicament. It defines how, why, and in what way he or she is ill."[10]

Nowadays we are challenged to find a place where clinical technologies do not silence the patients' voices and do not erase the individuality of each of the participants in the patient's journey. The plot in which the patient is situated demands of all caregivers the ability to respond as readers of that narrative.

Our narrative medicine platform will ensure that the patient's narrative is integrated into therapy itself, opening up silenced or non-existent dialogue space. The doubts, the fears and the expectations of the sick person can be registered and family members or caregivers, with whom the patient wants to share information, may enter these spaces, or in some of the rooms of this digital house. Prescriptions may include narratives of other patients who have shared their stories through this platform, as well as websites with valid scientific information. Therefore, therapy will not only be pharmacological or surgical, but also narrative, with the use of shared stories and with the opportunity provided to each patient to register their own diary. A semantic analysis software enables the signalling of patients who need to be seen by their doctors sooner than previously planned. Patients' and relatives' narratives allow for the tracking of significant changes in disease progression and in their own illness experience, thus precluding the patient and caregivers from feeling isolated. Moreover, the parallel chart registered on this platform by clinicians can direct their attention to alternative vantage points they can adopt when taking care of one particular patient.

---

10   Brian Hurwitz and Trisha Greenhalgh, "Why Study Narrative." *BMJ* 318 (1999): 48.

3   Final Remarks

Narrative-based digital platforms help to shift the focus to the patient and not only to the disease and allow doctors, nurses, social workers, and therapists to improve the effectiveness of care by developing the capacity for attention, reflection, representation and affiliation with patients and colleagues.

As Clandinin et al. have concluded in their study on the efficacy of narrative reflective practice strategy, the parallel chart process, with residents in family medicine and internal medicine, developing narrative competencies and reflecting narratively allow medical professionals to: "become more conscious of who they are in the physician-patient encounter; have their practices changes; recognize how they have changed over time and develop affiliation with that patients and colleagues."[11]

Texts like *The Storyteller* disturb our fantasy, and this is precisely what medical students need, what health professionals need, in order to reach the transperspectivity that is essential to keep track of our humanness:

> With narrative competence, physicians can reach and join their patients in illness, recognize their own personal journeys through medicine, acknowledge kinship with and duties toward other health care professionals, and inaugurate consequential discourse with the public about health care. By bridging the divides that separate physicians from patients, themselves, colleagues, and society, narrative medicine offers fresh opportunities for respectful, empathic, and nourishing medical care.[12]

We firmly believe that the interaction between Medicine and Narrative is an example for other social and educational practices that recognize the place of Humanities as an integral part of true knowledge in the service of man—one that is integrative and liberating, allowing for the recognition of our own vulnerability: "We're a pine needle before a fire, we're a speck of dirt before an earthquake, we're a drop of dew before a storm, dear friend."[13]

---

11   Jean Clandinin et al., "Learning Narratively: Resident Physicians' Experiences of a Parallel Chart Process." *Internet Journal of Medical Education* 1.1 (2010). 9, viewed 25 October 2016, http://ispub.com/IJME/1/1/12898.2009.

12   Rita Charon, "Narrative Medicine: A Model for Empathy, Reflection, Profession, and Trust," *JAMA* 286.15 (2001): 1897.

13   José Luís Peixoto, *Blank Gaze* (London: Bloomsbury Publishing, 2007), 81.

Bibliography

Anderson, Charles, and Martha Montello. "The Reader's Response and Why It Matters in Biomedical Ethics." In *Stories Matter: The Role of Narrative in Medical Ethics*, edited by Rita Charon and Martha Montello, 85–94. New York: Routledge, 2002.

Arendt, Hannah. *The Human Condition*. Chicago and London: The University of Chicago Press, 1958.

Berlinger, Nancy. "Resolving Harmful Mistakes: Is There a Role for Forgiveness?" *Virtual Mentor American Medical Association Journal of Ethics* 13.9 (2011): 647–654.

Blustein, Jeffrey. "On Taking Responsibility for One's Past." *Applied Philosophy* 17.1 (2000): 1–19.

Charon, Rita. "Narrative Medicine: A Model for Empathy, Reflection, Profession, and Trust." *JAMA* 286.15 (2001): 1897–1902.

Charon, Rita. *Narrative Medicine: Honoring the Stories of Illness*. Oxford: Oxford University Press, 2006.

Charon, Rita, and Martha Montello, ed. *Stories Matter: The Role of Narrative in Medical Ethics*. New York: Routledge, 2002.

Clandinin, D. Jean, Marie T Cave, Andrew Cave, Alan Thomson, and Hedy Bach. "Learning Narratively: Resident Physicians' Experiences of a Parallel Chart Process." *Internet Journal of Medical Education* 1.1. 2010. Viewed 25 October 2016. http://ispub.com/IJME/1/1/12898.

Frank, Arthur. W. *The Wounded Storyteller: Body, Illness and Ethics*, 2nd edition. Chicago and London: University of Chicago Press, 1995.

Frank, Arthur. W. *Letting Stories Breathe: A Socio-Narratology*. Chicago: The University of Chicago Press, 2010.

Hurwitz, Brian, and Trisha Greenhalgh, "Why Study Narrative." *BMJ* 318 (1999): 48–50.

Klitzman, Robert. *When Doctors Become Patients*. Oxford and New York: Oxford University Press, 2008.

Jurecic, Ann. *Illness as Narrative*. Pittsburgh: Pittsburgh University Press, 2012.

Peixoto, José Luís. *Blank Gaze*. London: Bloomsbury Publishing, 2007.

Picoult, Jodi. *The Storyteller*. London: Hodder & Stoughton, 2013.

Ricoeur, Paul. *Oneself as Another*. Translated by Kathleen Blamey. Chicago and London: The University of Chicago Press, 1992.

Ricoeur, Paul. *Le Juste*. Paris: Éditions Esprit, 1995.

Ricoeur, Paul, "Sanction, réabilitation, pardon." *Le Juste*, 193–208. Paris: Éditions Esprit, 1995.

Ricoeur, Paul. *Memory, History, Forgetting*. Translated by Kathleen Blamey and David Pellauer. Chicago: The University of Chicago Press, 2004.

Ricoeur, Paul, "The Difficulty to Forgive." In *Memory, Narrativity, Self and the Challenge to Think God: The reception within Theology of the Recent Work of Paul Ricoeur,* edited by Maureen Junker-Kenny and Peter Kenny, 6–16. New York and London: Transactions Publishers, 2004.

CHAPTER 9

Keeping Track of Humanness in the Novel
Never Let Me Go: Why Telling Matters

Susana Teixeira Magalhães

1   The Power of the Myth of Perfection

Stories about tragedies told in paintings and literary texts recall past events
that demand our current compromise not to allow the same kind of deeds to
take place, while opening a whole world of possibilities in the future. The suffering of the past can thus be redeemed by the promise not to let such deeds
happen again, or it can be deprived of its meaning and forgotten. Either way,
there is a whole world of possibilities into which human beings are born, since,
as Arendt reminds us, each birth is a new beginning:

> It is in the nature of beginning' – she claims – 'that something new is
> started which cannot be expected from whatever may have happened
> before. This character of startling unexpectedness is inherent in all
> beginnings.[1]

Never Let Me Go, a novel by Kazuo Ishiguro, makes us experience a world of
closure, of impossibility, predictability and silence, where each birth cannot
mean a new beginning, being instead a moment of repetition, mimicry, fab-
rication. It is a novel set up in a world where the ideal of a perfect and long-
lasting human being does not work any longer as a constant guiding light for
all human actions, within the gap between the ideal itself and reality.

Perfection first appeared in human imagination, before it was worked out
as a concept. In many cultures, this idea is presented as a myth, the myth of
origins. The terrestrial paradise of Christian-Jewish culture, the platonic myth
of the exiled soul and the Indian idea of the cosmic egg imply a lost primitive
wholeness at the origin of the world. It is as if mankind had already lived in
a golden age, being perfection understood as the quality of a self-fulfilled being that lingers identical to himself/herself. However, reality in the empirical

---

1   Arendt, *The Human Condition*, 177–178.

© KONINKLIJKE BRILL NV, LEIDEN, 2019 | DOI:10.1163/9789004386563_011

world is always changing and individuals' fulfilment is a never-ending story. The imaginary perfection underlying so many myths implies a stable subject, who does not have to go through a hard perfection process. According to Jean Ladriére, the myth has two main functions, which make it a fundamental stage in the human understanding of the world: first, it provides a pedagogy of transgression, since it requires a transgression of the empirical reality in order to imagine a perfect and whole human being from the time of his/her appearance – this is the reason why the myth was and has been the not totally overcome past of Philosophy and Science. It is worth noticing that Science improves through models that transgress the visible and apparent world. On the other hand, it works as pedagogy of the world creation in various stages, but it does so as if the world and mankind were already completely fulfilled, as if their task was nothing else except to act in a repetitive way, according to their own nature. Moreover, since the human being is aware of the fact that his/her own life does not match the original perfection, the myth must also tell about the event or the fall that led to the disappearance of this world of the origins. From our rational point of view, the myth discloses the need human beings have to think of their existence as a process that developed from a perfect model, as if they had to regain a lost paradise. This is why the myth of origins usually identifies with an eschatological one, in which the human subject regains the lost perfection. One can say that our existence is based both on the idea of the perfect mythical origins and the ideal of a regained perfection. Since the myth is at the basis of Reason, one wonders whether the scientific idea of an immortal and perfect human being can stem from the mythical ideal of a totally fulfilled being. It should be noticed that an ideal is by its own nature something that one cannot completely achieve, working instead as a constant guiding light for all human actions, within the gap between the ideal itself and reality. Whenever this gap is overridden and disrespected, human beings, and even science, can fall prey to the power of the myth. In this case, the ideal no longer works as the guiding light, but as an obsession one must accomplish at all costs.

In the world portrayed in the novel *Never Let Me Go*, this gap has already been overridden and disrespected, making us, the readers, understand what this violation of boundaries means for humanity and science. The love story between Kathy H. and Tommy D. draws us into the plot as we sense from the beginning that something odd looms ahead outside the boarding school Hailsham, located in the English countryside, the place where these characters belong to (even after leaving it). Though we are only told on pages 79 and 80 about the closed future of Hailsham students treated as merely medical by-products used to harvest organs for the benefit of the human population, we can actually read right from the start between what we are told and not told, much like what happens at Hailsham according to one of the teachers/ guardians, Miss Lucy: 'You were brought into this world for a purpose, and your futures, all of them, have been decided.'[2]

Action and nature, ethos and bios interact in a new way, which makes the ethos invade the field of bios, manipulating it according to its desires. In the world portrayed by Ishiguro's novel, human will can intervene in areas that have been out of human reach up till now, which requires thorough reflection upon the limits of such human actions. This is the field of a new myth – the myth of man's self-constitution – that tell us the narrative of humanity aiming to immerse all its bios within its ethos, self-making itself as purely rational. The respect for nature implies ethical limits to human action; but who should impose these limits? Divine intervention is not the answer, because the fundamentals for respecting biological nature are provided by the possibility of self-destruction by human beings. Why is not self-destruction one of the possibilities provided to human beings? It is a fact that human freedom always looms in the human horizon, in the same way that suicide lingers as an alternative way left open to our free will. However, the fact that self-destruction is always open to humanity discloses the preference for life as a kind of a priori evidence: it is better to live rather than not to live; existing is good; in principle, it is better to exist rather than not to exist. Existence is here understood as all the dimensions that make life authentically human – the dimensions that cloned life seems to be deprived from.

Miss Lucy's truth and her attempt to reveal to the cloned students living at Hailsham their real nature, from which there is no escape, assumes that, against all odds, these clones are not faceless and nameless, carrying instead unique names, faces and personalities. They are the Other that demands Miss Lucy's revelation, that explains our painfully hidden wish that their future could be different, that Kathy and Tommy could actually get a deferral and live longer. We even get impatient with the passivity of the main characters who obey the rules at Hailsham, later do exactly what is expected from them at the Cottages, carry on as Carers and finally as donors until they complete their cycle. The boundaries set up at Hailsham, that no student should cross, define the borders between the enclosed world of clones and the free world of the human beings living out there. In spite of all these strict boundaries, the humanity of the clones themselves is constantly sticking out, as if, despite all

---

2   Kazuo Ishiguro, *Never Let Me Go* (London: Faber and Faber, 2005), 79–80.

the efforts to keep them inside the labs, the boarding school, the Cottages, the hospitals, they end up being visibly human.

2   Narrative and Suffering: Why Telling Matters

Miss Lucy's story works in the same route but in the opposite direction of illness stories. In *The Wounded Storyteller*, Arthur W. Frank points out that 'illness narratives are wrecked because their present is not what the past was supposed to lead up to, and the future is scarcely thinkable.'[3] In the wounded world of *Never Let Me Go*, the present is tied up to the past and the future of each clone is inscribed in the moment of their creation, according to a programme that commodifies and instrumentalizes them. In spite of this difference, both illness stories and the story told by Miss Lucy have a dual function: to restore an order that the interruption fragmented and to tell the truth that the interruptions will continue. In the case of illness, the coherent sense of life is disrupted by disease and it can only be regained by telling the story of this particular experience, by restoring memory, by creating 'the memory structure that will contain the gist of the story for the rest of our lives. Talking is remembering.'[4] The person who becomes ill is not only interrupted by disease, but also in speech, schedule, sleep, solvency and these interruptions make others perceive you as interruptible. By telling the story of one's illness, individuals assume responsibility for their witness role and demand others to be the witnesses of their witnessing. The act of witnessing implies being true instead of telling what the others want to hear: 'This truth will trouble you, but in the end, you cannot be free without it, because you know it already; your body knows it already.'[5] Miss Lucy's narrative refuses silence and denial and, although her story is uncomfortable for Kathy, Tom, Ruth and the other students who listen to her, the truth is that they already knew it, their bodies knew it. Miss Lucy's version of their world restores the supposed order by revealing the truth that no future lies ahead except for the one that is supposed to be.

Kathy, the narrator of *Never Let Me Go*, whose eyes guide us into the plot, tells a story that is not only a memoir, but also a narrative from which a self is born, thus contradicting the logical assumption that in the case of clones the subject is already given and nothing can be learned. By telling about her life

---

3   Arthur W. Frank, *The Wounded Storyteller: Body, Illness and Ethics*, 2nd edition (Chicago and London: University of Chicago Press, 1995), 55.
4   Ibid., 61.
5   Ibid., 63.

as a clone she escapes partly from the cloned condition of isolation, empti-
ness, shadows, setting up the relationship that must exist whenever there is a
teller and a listener. Kathy, the storyteller, makes us look into the novel's question: what makes us human? In the territory of illness and caregiving the same
question is posed whenever the issue of dehumanized health service is raised
and whenever we have to face serious, chronic, and/or fatal illness. Kathy and
her friends Tom and Ruth are secluded form plurality, the human condition
that according to Hannah Arendt is necessary for human action, which might
explain the reactions and not the actions expected from the students at Hailsham and later from the veterans at the Cottages:

> There was, incidentally, something I noticed about these veteran couples
> at the Cottages – something Ruth, for all her close study of them, failed to
> spot – and this was how so many of their mannerisms were copied from
> the television.[6]

Works of art and motherly love are carefully overlooked at the boarding school,
thus precluding any trace of humanity. The drawings made by the students,
and strongly motivated by the guardians, are taken by a character called Madame to the so called Art Gallery, not to exhibit them, but to analyse them in
order to check if clones have a human soul after all. By taking these works of
Art away, society wants to ensure that, in spite of all the evidence of humanness in the Hailsham students, no trace of creativity, no sign of freedom will be
left behind. In *The Future of Human Nature*, Habermas points out that 'the fact
that this natural fate, this past before our past, so to speak, is not at our human
disposal seems to be essential for our awareness of freedom'.[7]

Habermas considers that genetically modified human beings and clones
are deprived of a future of their own, being unable to rebel against what was
decided before their existence started. What is important to underline about
The Future of Human Nature is the idea that human intervention in the nature
of humanity changes the ethical self-understanding of the species in an irre-
versible and unpredictable way. *Never Let Me Go* unveils some of the possible
consequences of this attempt to work out the myth of human perfection in the
here and now. Madame cries when she sees Kathy pretending to hold a baby
in her arms while listening to the song *Never Let me Go* by Judy Bridgewater
and Miss Lucy bursts out drawing for not being allowed to tell Tommy and the

---

6   Ishiguro, *Never Let Me Go*, 119.
7   Jürgen Habermas. *The Future of Human Nature*. Translated by W. Rehg, M. Pensky, and H. Beis-
    ter (Cambridge: Polity, 2003), 59.

other students that their drawings are not valued per se, but only as part of a social experiment to verify the humanness of clones.

Kathy is between two worlds, seeing from inside the clones' environment and reaching out to the world where the so called normal people live by narrating about her life. Entropy is what best describes the instrumentalization of these characters, always surrounded by fences, glass windows, windscreens. Seclusion is reinforced by the clones mimicry, particularly in the case of Ruth, who tends to replicate the gestures and the words of the veterans, the older clones at the Cottages. In spite of silence and of all the simulation environment surrounding these characters, the fact is that they give us clues to what makes us human. Their humanity is perceived and reaffirmed by their capacity to love, to act for the others, to feel compassion, and to be able to tell about it. No matter how instrumentalized they are perceived by the rest of the society, they are more than a shadow, which might explain the unnamed fear of the normal people towards clones and the symmetrical fear of the clones towards the world out there:

> So, you're waiting, even if you don't quite know it, waiting for the moment when you realise that you are really different to them. That there are people out there, like Madame, who don't hate you or wish you any harm, but who nevertheless shudder at the very thought of you – of how you were brought into this world and why – and who dread the idea of your hand brushing against theirs.[8]

Kathy's narrative reveals what happens when individuals are commodified and their stories are silenced: all the possible futures are cut and hope is deconstructed. It also underlines the unsuccessful attempt to efface the self of those instrumentalized, because their humanity will squeeze out of the borders imposed by science and technology. *Never Let Me Go* is more about how we frame our narratives and those of the others, than about cloning; it is more about the way human beings try to outdistance mortality by rendering illness transitory; its focus is more on the chaotic lack of coherence when vulnerability, futility and impotence dominate oneself; it is more about having a voice of one's own while going on a journey that becomes a quest. Restitution narratives promise a safe landing, and do not integrate suffering and unexpected failures. This is the narrative that lies at the bottom of the cloning programme, being the clones the instrument that ensures the mortality will be outdistanced. Below

---

8   Ishiguro, *Never Let Me Go*, 36.

the surface of normality, there lies chaos which is visible in Tommy's tantrums, Miss Lucy's furious scrawling over a page with a pencil, Madame's fear of Hailsham students, our own awareness of our powerlessness to keep Kathy, Ruth and Tommy together, to never let them go. The quest narrative is the story told by Kathy, who tells her own story and integrates the suffering by perceiving illness as a journey, a motif that is present in this novel by the constant reference to the boundaries that one should not cross. Kathy, Tommy and Ruth know the limits to their walks around Hailsham and the Cottages, and in spite of their freedom to run away, they do not break the rules, being thus always moving out and always walking back to the same place. In a world without the family structure, the guardians at Hailsham and the school itself stand for the umbilical cord that provide a beginning for the narrative identity built by each of the main characters, mainly by Kathy. The place where they are and the place where we, readers, might be, are for Kathy the origin that explains who each of us is. Place and time intersect on the roads that the characters are eager to explore, which is all the more ironic and meaningful if we bear in our minds that they are going nowhere. The Norfolk trip stands as the most important journey, since it is both a forward-looking journey, in search for Ruth's possible, the original human being from whom she was copied, and a backward-looking journey on the shadows of Hailsham. In the end, Kathy's tape of Judy Bridgewater, *Songs of Darkness*, is found, not recovered, because, unlike the social image of clones and empty vessels, the things they own can still keep their singularity and the tape found at Norfolk is not the original. The woman Kathy, Tommy and Ruth thought could be Ruth's possible is not the one they were looking for, so the trip to Norfolk changes the Hailsham illusion of a possible future: 'On that journey home, with the darkness setting in over those long empty roads, it felt like the three of us were close again and I didn't want anything to come along and break that mood' (181). But the mood is broken and their programme is completed, after they go through the experience of being caregivers and then donators. What is striking about the period as caregivers, is the twist that Ishiguro introduces in the plot, because solitude, powerlessness, the feeling that one is giving the other a life worth living, even if only for some days or weeks, is common to all caregivers. If these clones share the same feelings with other caregivers, then here could lie the answer to the question 'What is it that makes us human?'

3   Final Remarks

In order to keep one's word, there must be a Self and Another, because without the experience of recognition (that is indeed an experience of mutual recognition), self-attestation is not possible. In *Narrative Medicine: Honouring the stories of illness*, Rita Charon relates 'the medical impulse toward replication and universality' (that condemns the characters of Ishiguro's novel to instrumentalization) to the muted *doctor's realization of the singularity and creativity of their acts of observation and description.*

Hence, the replica of clones that this novel confronts us with is already here, not in the labs, not in the actual cloning process, but in the impersonal, science-based doctor-patient relations that demand bridges to decrease the divides present in health care. These bridges, that narrative skills enable between 'doctor and patient or nurse and patient, are echoed and recapitulated in collegial relations between doctor and nurse, and in the even wider reflective communitas between patients in their neighbourhoods and the health professionals who serve them'.[9] Therefore, there is a web of relations that improve with the focus on the individual and the singular, instead of focusing on the statistics and the universal. Turning to narrative and *letting stories breathe*[10] in healthcare, implies setting up solid foundations, which can be found in Philosophy, Ethics and Literature.

Like many illness stories that restore the public visibility of death, Kathy's story borrows its authority from death and lingers beyond the expected death of the narrator. It is a story that will surely continue in other stories, in the so called web of stories that Arthur W. Frank quotes from Walter Benjamin's *The Storyteller*: 'Each story weaves threads that are original in that person's experience. Yet, everything that is said carries the resonance of previous stories (...).'[11]

Ishiguro's story warns us against the loss of individuality and singularity in a fabricated world, which resonates significantly in the territory of caregiving. The web of stories, which this novel makes part of, should be preserved, so that radical hope can be offered to those who suffer and to those who care.

Bibliography

Anderson, Charles, and Martha Montello, "The Reader's Response and Why It Matters in Biomedical Ethics." In *Stories Matter: The Role of Narrative in Medical Ethics*, edited by Rita Charon and Martha Montello, 85–94. New York: Routledge, 2002.

---

9   Rita Charon. *Narrative Medicine: Honoring the Stories of Illness* (Oxford: Oxford University Press, 2006), 229.

10   Arthur W. Frank. *Letting Stories Breathe: A Socio-Narratology* (Chicago: The University of Chicago Press, 2010).

11   Frank, *The Wounded Storyteller*, 220.

Arendt, Hannah. *The Human Condition*. Chicago and London: The University of Chicago Press, 1958.

Berlinger, Nancy, "Resolving Harmful Mistakes: Is There a Role for Forgiveness?" *Virtual Mentor American Medical Association Journal of Ethics* 13.9 (2011): 647–654.

Blustein, Jeffrey, "On Taking Responsibility for One's Past." *Applied Philosophy* 17.1 (2000): 1–19.

Charon, Rita. *Narrative Medicine: Honoring the Stories of Illness*. Oxford: Oxford University Press, 2006.

Frank, Arthur. W. *The Wounded Storyteller: Body, Illness and Ethics*, 2nd edition. Chicago and London: University of Chicago Press, 1995.

Frank, Arthur. W. *Letting Stories Breathe: A Socio-Narratology*. Chicago: The University of Chicago Press, 2010.

Habermas, Jürgen. *The Future of Human Nature*. Translated by W. Rehg, M. Pensky, and H. Beister. Cambridge: Polity, 2003.

Heidegger, Martin. *Contributions to Philosophy*. Translated by Richard Rojcewicz, and Daniela Vallega-Neu. Indiana: Indiana University Press, 2012.

Ishiguro, Kazuo. *Never Let Me Go*. London: Faber and Faber, 2005.

Ladrière, Jean. *Éléments de critique des sciences et de cosmologie*. Louvain: Université Catholique, 1996.

Matthiessen, Francis Otto. *American Renaissance: Art and Expression in the Age of Emerson and Whitman*. New York: Oxford University Press, 1972

Ricoeur, Paul. *Oneself as Another*. Translated by Kathleen Blamey. Chicago and London: The University of Chicago Press, 1992.

Ricoeur, Paul. *The Course of Recognition*. London: Harvard University Press, 2005.

Ricoeur, Paul. *Philosophie de la volonté: le volontaire et l'involontaire*. Paris: Éditions de Points, 2009.

CHAPTER 10

Incendies: Singing, Silencing and Writing as Healing Strategies

Davina Marques

Resistance for me is a mission
and part of this mission is the talking about it.[1]
SOHA BECHARA

∴

1   Wadji Mouawad

Wadji Mouawad (1968-) is a Lebanese-Canadian actor, director, translator and playwright. This is his possible short biography:

> Mouawad has lived with the tension between personal agency and un-stoppable world forces since his childhood, which he has summarized as "one war, two exiles, and a death." Born in Beirut, he was six when the Lebanese Civil War erupted in April 1975.
>
> Hundreds of thousands fled the country, including Mouawad and his family. They emigrated to Paris. In 1983, unable to renew their French visas, they moved again, this time to Quebec. Mouawad's mother died from cancer a year later.[2]

Considered the theatre's most impressive new voice in the last decade, he has produced intensively since 1992.[3] I first heard of him because of the film *Incendies*, by Denis Villeneuve (2010), based on Mouawad's homonymous play,

---

1   Jayce Salloum, "untitled part 1: everything and nothing," (France/Canada, video), 2001, accessed March 23, 2016, https://vimeo.com/71401594.
2   Dan Rubin, "Wadji Mouawad – At Home with Words," *Words on Plays 2011/12 season* vol. XVIII 4 (2012): 4.
3   "Wadji Mouawad – Bibliographie," *Wadji Mouawad*, accessed June 24, 2016, http://www.wajdimouawad.fr/wajdi-mouawad/bibliographie.

which was later translated to English with the title *Scorched*. This play alone has had more than a hundred productions in several languages, Portuguese included, with a strongly acclaimed staged play in Brazil.

According to the text that he writes in the introduction to the published play, Mouawad wrote *Incendies* over eight months, during a process of rehearsing it, working with actors.

In interviews, Mouawad has also mentioned the fact that the main character, Nawal Marwan, was inspired by the Lebanese political activist Soha Bechara. This is how he presents the theme of war, which traverses the story:

> War is where the collective and the intimate collide. My question is how to be happy personally when the collective isn't working. The history of our inner lives is as complex as our collective history. In the stories that I tell, I ask the questions: How far can we go? How do we console? How do we find safety?[4]

The author leads us on a journey into an unnamed land in the Middle East, and it involves us readers in stories of hatred, wars, fights, and incredibly constant love.

In this paper I intend to explore a scene from the play (performance), one from the text (the published version of the play) and a sequence from the film by Denis Villeneuve. My objective is to highlight different aspects of healing for the character, while, at the same time, to bring forth the idea that art heals and we, the people who appreciate or get involved in it, like patients, also heal – from daily misfortunes, pains, abandonment, and problems.

2   A Scene from the Play – Silencing

Different productions use distinct approaches in their plays. As we read about the sketches envisioned in the play release, and as we watch the Canadian production online in comparison with the Brazilian conception, we can get a grasp of the unlimited possibilities.

I have discussed the issue of adapting literature to film before.[5] Theoretically based on contemporary French philosophy, by Gilles Deleuze, I argue that fabulation is an interesting approach to compare different arts or works

---

4 Rubin, "Wadji Mouawad," 6.
5 Davina Marques, "Entre Literatura, Cinema e Filosofia: Miguilim nas Telas" (Ph. D., Universidade de São Paulo, 2013).

of art.[6] The objective here, however, is not to compare productions or adaptations of *Incendies*. My intention is to approach the play and analyse the plot as a project of healing, observing how the main character, Nawal Marwan, is able to deal with extremely difficult situations in her life. Therefore, I would like to start with a recorded scene from the French Canadian version of the play.[7]

Incendies tell the story of Nawal Marwan.

There was love in the beginning, and it was destroyed right then. A Muslim and a Christian have no permission to hope for love in the territory of the Gods. No mercy; no God for their mercy. Vows were exchanged. She told the man she loved: "No matter what happens, come what may, I will love you forever. I will always love you."[8]

As they were not meant to be together, the young man was killed. Nawal was left alone, single, and pregnant. Shame and dirt would be brought upon her family's name if anyone ever found out. Her only way out: to give the baby away after he was born.

The baby is still with her when a new promise is made, now to her son: "I will find you again. No matter what happens, come what may, I will love you forever. I will always love you."[9]

And the child was taken from her arms, the same arms which had been forbidden to embrace her chosen loved one.

Silencing kept Nawal sane then. What could she say if she had no voice?

After one long year of seeing her granddaughter's silent sadness, Nazira found herself in the last moments of life (this is the scene I highlight from the play). She called Nawal to tell her that there was hope. Nawal should not give in. She should be brave and work hard: she should leave the village and learn how to read, how to write. It was her only chance to be freed from the web of hatred that their family had turned into. They had hated each other so long; her grandmother said that she, Nawal, might also leave hatred behind, as heritage, if she did not do anything about it. There was such a history of misery in their lives. By educating herself, Nawal would be able to escape from that legacy of suffering. Her grandmother made her promise that Nawal would learn how to read and then she would come back and write her name on her

6 Gilles Deleuze and Félix Guattari, *Essays Critical and Clinical*, trans. Daniel W. Smith and Michael A. Greco (London; New York: Verso, 1998).

7 Dorothée Duplan. "Extrait d'Incendies de Wajdi Mouawad," (video), June 10, 2013, accessed October 15, 2015. https://www.youtube.com/watch?v=AbLpJ6CLTXk.

8 Wadji Mouawad, *Incêndios*, trans. Ângela Leite Lopes (Rio de Janeiro: Cobogó, 2013), 46. [author's own translation into English]

9 Mouawad, *Incêndios*, 47. [author's own translation into English]

tombstone. Her grandmother had kept all her promises; and she should do the same. Spoken words are powerful. Keeping your word means a lot.

Nawal promised to do so, and she did leave the village after burying her grandmother. She had learned the importance of rising above misery. Nawal loved her grandmother; she owed her. She also wanted to find her son.

When she returned to the village, years later, to fulfil her promise, Nawal said that she was ready then to start looking for her child, the one she had promised to love no matter what, forever.

Silencing had been a way to deal with suffering and having to accept what her family wanted for her. Silencing was going to be a resource again in the future: silence became a resource to survive later in her life. The story starts with a notary delivering Nawal's last wishes to two young adults – her children:

> Bury me naked
> Bury me without a coffin
> No clothing
> No praying
> Face to the ground [...]
> No stone will be placed on my tomb
> No name will be recorded
> No epitaph for those who don't keep their promises.
> And one promise was not kept.
> No epitaph for those who keep the silence.
> And silence was kept.[10]

Jeanne and Simon, Nawal's children, received one letter each after she died. Simon was supposed to hand the letter he received to his brother. Jeanne's was destined to her father. Only after they had delivered these letters would Nawal be able to be honoured with a tombstone with her name engraved on it.

The problem was they didn't even know they had a father; they had no idea they had a brother. The tension of the exquisite request sets us on the uneasiness of the strange situation.

Nawal had been silent for five years before she died. Jeanne, her daughter, decided to understand why and to do as she was told. Simon resisted.

Can silence heal?

---

10   Mouawad, *Incêndios*, 25–27. [author's own translation into English]

3   An Excerpt from the Film – Singing

Nawal started her journey. And in the attempt to find her child, the protagonist found herself in war. She became politically involved – basically in order to survive –, and killed an important leader. She was taken as a political prisoner.

In prison, she became a giant, in Deleuzian terms: she became *the woman-who-sings*. She was beaten, tortured, raped, over and over again, but they could not break her. In this period of her life they could not silence her. She sang in prison. She sang to console herself and her fellow prisoners. She sang while others were being tortured. And it enraged brutal men around her. Nawal became a myth.

How does one become a myth? What makes one a martyr?

When he tried to understand the characteristics of the stories he liked, Gilles Deleuze came up with the idea of fabulation. One of the elements of fabulating is exactly myth-making or the creation of a giant. Art resists death, servitude, intolerance, shame, as it fabulates giants, Deleuze argues. The artist "has seen something in life that is too great, too unbearable also [...]. But this something is also the source or breath that supports them through the illnesses of the lived (what Nietzsche called health)."[11]

This part of the plot is based on the life story of Soha Bechara (1967-), the activist who is the best-known political prisoner of the Lebanese Civil War. She spent ten years of her life in the Khiam prison, which was condemned by the United Nations for its inhumane conditions. She has spoken about the cruel practices she suffered in her books. She was threatened sexually despite the fact that she has never mentioned rape. Mouawad's character wasn't so "lucky," and gave birth in prison.

Bechara described "singing in solitary – next to the room where prisoners were being tortured – and hoping her voice would give others hope."[12]

Silencing is no remedy in this situation. Singing becomes a way to resist suffering, humiliation, and pain.

Can a song heal?

---

11   Gilles Deleuze and Félix Guattari, *What is Philosophy?*, trans. Janis Tomlinson and Graham Burchell III (Columbia: Columbia University Press, 2014), 172–173. See also Ronald Bogue, *Deleuzian Fabulation and the Scars of History* (Edinburgh: Edinburgh University Press, 2010).

12   Kate Goldstein, "A Life of Resistance – A Brief Biography of Soha Bechara," *Words on Plays 2011/12 season* vol. XVIII 4 (2012): 38.

4   An Excerpt from the Text – Writing

It is difficult to write about this play without spoiling the reading for others. It is composed as a big puzzle, with flash-backs that fill in missing pieces. Nawal's daughter had to go to her mother's country with nothing but her personal documents, a photograph and a jacket with a number 72 on the back – and she had no idea what it meant.

I must declare, however, that knowing the whole story does not prevent the tears from coming every time I see the film or play and read the text again. The story is powerful, the ending is incredible; I strongly advise everyone to read or see it.

The play starts and ends with an act of writing. There is an unexpected will in the beginning, which reveals to Jeanne and Simon that their father and brother live; and the last pages of the play offer us the reading of three letters. The two mentioned in the beginning, meant to be delivered to Nawal's children's father and brother; and another one, meant for her children, Jeanne and Simon, to be read only after they are able to find their unknown father and brother.

The "contradictory intertwined leitmotifs" in this plot are the necessity to keep the silence and then the need to break it; and the sacred nature of promises.[13] Nawal had promised to find her child. She felt she had failed to do so. She kept the secret.

Five years before her death, she was a witness in court and then something changed her life once again and she was forced to do something about it.

Nawal stopped talking. She could not pronounce another word. It made Jeanne and Simon suffer from being shut off.

Nevertheless, she was not really only silent then: she was writing. She was resisting.

Her drama was so tremendously incredible, unbearable, that she had to protect herself. On the other hand, she understood she was going to be able to bring her children closer, while making them learn about who she really was.

They found their father, their brother.

In her final letter she asked Jeanne and Simon if they were laughing, if they were crying. She did not advise them to stop. She wrote that "Childhood is a knife struck in the throat," but Simon was able to pull it out. She told Jeanne that the women in their family "were tied in a web of anger"; it was necessary to break that web. It was necessary to reconstruct their fragmented story; slowly consoling each piece; healing every memory; slowly, as if in a lullaby.

---

13   Elizabeth F. Dahab, "Of Broken Promises and Mended Lives," in *Voices of Exile in Contemporary Canadian Francophone Literature* (Maryland: Lexington Books, 2011), 145.

She urged them to think of the beginning of their history back to the day when a young woman went back to her village to write her grandmother Nazira's name on her tombstone. And then she adds her final request:

> When asked about your life story,
> Tell people that your story goes back in time to a day
> When a girl went back to her home village
> in order to engrave a name on her grandmother's tombstone.
> There your story begins.
> Jeanne, Simon,
> Why didn't I tell you?
> There are truths that can only be discovered.
> You have opened the envelopes, you have broken the silence.
> Write my name on a stone
> and place it on my tomb.
>   Your mother[14]

Can a letter heal?

5   Living as a Patient and Healing

The whole point of the journey taken by Nawal is to break the thread, to escape the circle of hatred and avoid the misery of the life her family had to put up with, just as her grandmother had told her to do.

I have ended each section of this paper with a question: can silence, singing or a letter heal?

I like the concept of the artists as physicians, as symptomatologists – just like doctors and clinicians; storytelling in literature and cinema as a way to save lives.[15]

Art constantly offers us examples of possibilities to deal with our daily misfortunes, our pains, our feelings of abandonment, and our problems. In this sense it heals. It makes us go back to our own selves.

When the artists dive into chaos and return with red eyes, and work their ideas through the monuments they construct, we are offered a block of sensation, which moves the ones in contact with it.[16]

---

14   Mouawad, *Incêndios*, 132–133. [author's own translation into English]
15   Davina Marques and Fabiana Carelli, "Healing Representations in Literature and Cinema," in *Beyond Present Patient Realities: Collaboration, Care and Identity*, eds. Peter Bray and Ana Maria Borlescu (Oxford: Inter-Disciplinary Press, 2015), 35–47.
16   Deleuze and Guattari, *What is Philosophy?*, 2014.

"Be patient ... Nothing is more beautiful than being together."[17] Nawal understood that bonding was the way to break the thread of hatred and misery. In that sense, she has healed, and she has also healed her broken family – through singing, silencing and writing.

> *We have no boundaries.*
> *Our boundaries should be the love that continues forward.*[18]
> SOHA BECHARA

Bibliography

Bogue, Ronald. *Deleuzian Fabulation and the Scars of History*. Edinburgh: Edinburgh University Press, 2010.

Dahab, Elizabeth. *Voices of Exile in Contemporary Canadian Francophone Literature*. Maryland: Lexington Books, 2011.

Deleuze, Gilles and Félix Guattari. *Essays Critical and Clinical*. Translated by Daniel W. Smith and Michael A. Greco. London; New York: Verso, 1998.

Deleuze, Gilles and Félix Guattari. *What is Philosophy?* Translated by Janis Tomlinson and Graham Burchell III. Columbia: Columbia University Press, 2014.

Duplan, Dorothée. "Extrait d'Incendies de Wajdi Mouawad" (video). June 10, 2013. Accessed October 15, 2015. https://www.youtube.com/watch?v=AbLpJ6CLTXk.

Goldstein, Kate. "A Life of Resistance – A Brief Biography of Soha Bechara." *Words on Plays 2011/12 season* 18.4 (2012): 35–39.

Incendies. DVD. Directed by Denis Villeneuve. Toronto: Les Films Séville, 2010. DVD.

Marques, Davina. "Entre Literatura, Cinema e Filosofia: Miguilim nas Telas." Ph.D., Universidade de São Paulo, 2013.

Marques, Davina, and Fabiana Carelli. "Healing Representations in Literature and Cinema." In *Beyond Present Patient Realities: Collaboration, Care and Identity*, edited by Peter Bray and Ana Maria Borlescu, 35–47. Oxford: Inter-Disciplinary Press, 2015.

Mouawad, Wadji. *Incêndios*. Translated by Ângela Leite Lopes. Rio de Janeiro: Cobogó, 2013.

Mouawad, Wajdi. *Scorched*. Translated by Linda Gaboriau. Toronto: Playwrights Canada Press, 2010.

Rubin, Dan. "Wadji Mouawad – At Home with Words." *Words on Plays 2011/12 season* 18.4 (2012): 4–10.

Salloum, Jayce. "untitled part 1: everything and nothing" (video). 2001. Accessed March 23, 2016. https://vimeo.com/71401594.

---

17   Mouawad, *Incêndios*, 129.
18   "untitled part 1".

CHAPTER 11

A Postmodern Exploration of the Screened Dialogue between Past and Present and the Acceptance of Domestic Gender Performativity in Ventura Pons' *Barcelona (un mapa)* (2007)

Jytte Holmqvist

1 Introduction

This paper features an analysis of the postmodern elements in Pons' *Barcelona (un mapa)* (2007). In focus is the constant dialogue between past and present in the film partly achieved through interspersed sequences of real footage from Barcelona's past, which adds to the mosaic and also cartographic layout of the film, and, importantly, Pons' representation of gender performativity in a society and era where a man's need to explore the opposite gender by dressing the part also in the open is still not always readily embraced. Also highlighted is the tolerant relationship between a Catalan husband and wife and the ultimately circular narrative structure which enables Pons to end the film in a manner similar to the way in which it began.

In keeping with the film title, the paper additionally examines Pons' representation of Barcelona as a capital that can be mapped and spatially explored, the scenes depicting Barcelona's non-homogenous architecture, and the use of the cinematic photo-effect as a way to connect the pre-democratic past with the global present represented on screen.

Ever faithful to the Catalan region, language and culture, Pons has proven repeatedly that success can be achieved also by working in a minority language. In films where characters generally speak Catalan, their often problematic and strained relationships are highlighted while at the same time the cineaste paints a global image of Barcelona that reflects his awareness of concurrent urban developments. In the words of Jaume Martí-Olivella, "Ventura Pons is perhaps the only film-maker who has established a personal cinematic idiom about the city [of Barcelona], his own city."[1] Indeed, this becomes evident in

---

1 Jaume Martí-Olivella, "Catalan Cinema: An Uncanny Transnational Performance," *A Companion to Catalan Culture*, ed. Dominic Keown (Woodbridge, Suffolk: Tamesis, 2011), 200.

Pons' tendency to repeatedly use Barcelona as a metropolitan backdrop for his plots. In his oeuvre, Pons – steeped in a theatrical background – draws inspiration from novels or stage plays by prominent Catalan writers and playwrights such as Lluís-Anton Baulenas, Sergi Belbel, and Lluïsa Cunillé. The cinematic result is a number of theatrical elements, scenes where only a few characters converse at a time, and very direct dialogues that often have an almost visceral effect on the viewer.

Postmodern cinema has been defined as one that

> thrives on simulation (using comedy or pastiche to imitate former genres or styles), prefabrication (reworking what is already there rather than inventing materials), intertextuality (texts exist in relationship to other texts and are tissues of quotations from other texts) and bricolage (assemblage of works from eclectic sources).[2]

Adhering to these criteria, several of Pons' films can be regarded as cross-disciplinary as he establishes a connection between theatre and cinema. This is certainly the case in *Barcelona (un mapa)*, based on Cunillé's 2004 screenplay. The plot revolves around tenants told to vacate their flats in an apartment building in central Barcelona when ailing elderly landlord Ramon declares that he wishes to spend his remaining days alone with wife Rosa. As the tenants individually respond to the news we glimpse their personalities while at the same time Pons draws a seemingly fragmented yet ultimately complete portrait of the couple leasing the apartments. And what appears to be a film firmly set in the here and now turns out to be much more when the past is invited into the present through a number of cinematographic techniques.

2   Postmodern Elements and Urban Landmarks

Translated into English as *Barcelona, Map of Shadows*, this title remains faithful to the original Catalan title. The historical shadow play that we become witness to could mainly refer to the shadows from the Catalan past that linger in a visual narrative generally steeped in the global present (although in the final scene the great map of shadows that is *Barcelona (un mapa)* is also explained in more concrete terms). Apart from in these visual fragments, the

---

2   This excerpt from page 9 of Shohini Chaudhuri's book *Contemporary World Cinema: Europe, The Middle East, East Asia and South Asia* (2005) paraphrases Susan Hayward's *Cinema Studies: The Key Concepts* (London and New York: Routledge, 2000, second edition), 277–278, 283.

film's postmodernity is reflected in its pastiche or collage-like structure, with a deconstructionist *montage* at times considered "the primary form of post-modern discourse"[3] and which challenges a conventionally chronological time pattern in a nonlinear manner, and in lengthy dialogues where we get an in-sight into the mind of each character. Thus, a slow narrative pace and a focus on character development are favoured over external action. Pons' theatrical plot structure makes for a film that criss-crosses between past and present by way of regular flashbacks from times gone by and an opening scene featuring black and white footage of the decisive moment when Franco forces entered Barcelona unopposed in January 1939.[4] A postmodern, hybrid filmic text is cre-ated which visually interweaves different eras and where real footage is used to complement a fictive storyline set in a screened present.

In the film, Pons paints a disturbing yet realistic picture of a number of individuals whose lives in global Barcelona are impaired by their inability to fully embrace an urban environment that they neither fully recognise nor tolerate. Here, the postmodern architecture – at a time when it becomes "the norm to seek out 'pluralistic' and 'organic' strategies for approaching urban development as a 'collage' of highly differentiated spaces and mixtures"[5] contrasts starkly with the more classical architecture of old Barcelona. Mak-ing up the real, off-screen cityscape are more traditional buildings erected during Catalonia's periods of Romanticism, Neo-classicism and Historicism. Neo-Gothic elements also feature in the city architecture. A product of the post-moderniste[6] Catalan movement, Antoni Gaudí, whose Roman Catho-lic landmark La Sagrada Familia draws negative criticism in Pons' film, has left a baroque imprint on the urban landscape; with buildings often steeped in a ground-breaking modernity.[7] His unconventional, hitherto incomplete

---

3   David Harvey, *The Condition of Postmodernity: An Enquiry into the Origins of Cultural Change* (Oxford, England and Cambridge, Massachusetts: Blackwell, 1989), 51. Harvey here refers to Derrida.

4   Not surprisingly, the film has been called a "metaphor for the recent history of Catalo-nia." Barcelona (un mapa) 2007. *Cambridge Film Festival*, viewed 6 June, 2013, http://www.cambridgefilmfestival.org.uk/films/2012/barcelona

5   Harvey, *The Condition of Postmodernity: An Enquiry into the Origins of Cultural Change* (Oxford, England and Cambridge, Massachusetts: Blackwell, 1989), 40.

6   Arthur Terry stresses that "Catalan modernism – not to be confused with Spanish *mod-ernismo*, whose context is quite different – was above all an attempt to create a genuinely modern, European culture out of what was felt to be a purely local and regional one." "Catalan Literary *Modernisme* and *Noucentisme*: From Dissidence to Order," in *Spanish Cultural Studies. An Introduction: The Struggle for Modernity*, eds. Helene Graham and Jo Labanyi (New York: Oxford University Press, 1995), 55.

7   In David Mackay's words, "Catalan culture, always at the cross-roads of European move-ments, absorbed these tendencies through Gaudí, Domènech and Puig, reshaping their

cathedral has received mixed reviews from residents and visitors alike – and so it does also from the very film characters, some of whom scream at the pointy church in open rejection and disgust while, ironically, in the same breath sympathising with it by subjectifying and pitying it for being surrounded by other in their mind equally abominable, more recent, urban constructs.

The urban map referred to in Pons' movie title also becomes narratively and visually distinguishable in the cartographic layout of the film. It appears Pons has been guided by Sergei Eisenstein's view that "[f]ilm's undoubted ancestor ... is – architecture."[8] Thus, when set in the global present, the film becomes a city guide where protagonists walk us through the nocturnal streets, adding their personal commentary on the transformed space in heated dialogues where they express dissatisfaction with several urban landmarks. Apart from rejecting the Sagrada Familia, they also voice a desire to set fire to select buildings (an apparent reference is here made to a real fire at the Gran Teatre del Liceu, in 1994).[9] Whether or not Ramon – ex night porter at the Liceu Opera House and a husband with a penchant for crossdressing after being at once inspired and fascinated by female costume-change in the changing rooms at the Opera House – has in fact succeeded in igniting[10] this very theatre, as suggested at the end of the film, remains uncertain and is something left to the viewer's imagination.

---

contradictory aspects to produce the finest examples of national Modernist architecture: a Romantic architecture that, while harking back to an idealized medieval era, was free to respond to the functional requirements of a new mode, personally interpreted and popularly understood as being appropriate to the aspirations and self-image of a country that wished to express both its unique personality and its integral modernity." David Mackay, *Modern Architecture in Barcelona (1854–1939)* (UK: The University of Sheffield Printing Unit, 1985), 42.

8   – as cited by Giuliana Bruno in "Site-Seeing: Architecture and the Moving Image," *Wide Angle* 19.4 (1997): 8.

9   Resina remarks that "[i]f I were to choose a counterimage to the flaming arrow lighting the Olympic torch, it would be the sparks from welders setting the opera house on fire on January 31, 1994, just a year and a half after the Olympics. Watching the gaping crater of the Liceu, Barcelonans awoke from self-congratulatory enchantment to the cold reality of negligence." Joan Ramon Resina, *Barcelona's Vocation of Modernity: Rise and Decline of an Urban Image* (Stanford, California: Stanford University Press, 2008), 232.

10   With an additional link to Pedro Almodóvar, it has been noted that "[t]o burn something down it may also be necessary to build something new. It is a slow-paced film whose characters are full of surprises with a distinct similarity, however seemingly unlikely, to

3   Urban Dystopia

Barcelona (un mapa) highlights the complex relationship between the protagonists and their partly unrecognisable urban habitat. They experience a bewildering sense of *architorture*[11] and remain apprehensive towards buildings that are architecturally and aesthetically non-homogeneous and whose surface glamour reflects the sleek postmodern architecture of Barcelona; such as the 1957 Camp Nou stadium and the Torre Agbar skyscraper, erected in 2005. These modern constructs add a shiny gloss to a city with a troublesome past that still haunts the characters.[12] And thus, although there is constant communication between the protagonists in this metropolitan, semi-historical drama, they are all the more incapable of establishing a dialogue with their own city. With a clear Deleuzian reference made, Anton Pujol talks of a sense of deterritorialisation in the film, brought about by "nationalism, *Modernisme*," and "anarchism."[13] In our global era, this feeling of "un-belonging" and rootlessness also signifies the erosion and eventual collapse of any clear delimitations between culture and a specific place. Rather, in today's multicultural society urban space, in particular, has become more fluid and there is a loosening of cultural ties and boundaries which is reflected in Pons' film. This leads to a sense of alienation amongst his characters towards their architecturally experimental habitat. In a de-territorialized Deleuzian fashion, "[w]hen the cosmic connections of an endless line of the universe are severed," the result is the "emergence of a disoriented, disconnected space."[14] Specifically, in *Barcelona (un mapa)*, the protagonists are seemingly as disoriented in their post-Olympic environment as

       Almodóvar's universe." *Barcelona un mapa*, viewed 27 February 2013, http://andysfilm-world.blogspot.com.au/2008/12/barcelona-map-spain.html

11   This concept has been defined as a "sense of homelessness ... a primal sense of loss, a loss that has lost nothing, that has always already existed and that, like Baudrillard's simulacrum, has no origin or original, but underpins the very possibility of existence." David Sorfa, "Architorture: Jan Švankmajer and Surrealist Film," in *Screening the City*, eds. Mark Shiel and Tony Fitzmaurice (London and New York: Verso, 2003), 108.

12   According to Antonio Sánchez, "[f]iguratively speaking, it can be said that Barcelona's redevelopment has transformed the ailing modern city into a gigantic postmodern mirror reflecting an idealized image of itself to local and global audiences alike." Antonio Sánchez, "Barcelona's Magic Mirror: Narcissism or the Rediscovery of Public Space and Collective Identity?," in *Constructing Identity in Contemporary Spain: Theoretical Debates and Cultural Practice*, ed. Jo Labanyi (New York: Oxford University Press, 2002), 303.

13   Antón Pujol, "Ventura Pons's *Barcelona (un mapa)*: Trapped in the Crystal," *Studies in Hispanic Cinemas* 6, no. 1 (2009): 72.

14   Ronald Bogue, *Deleuze on Cinema* (London and New York: Routledge, 2003), 99.

Barcelona itself would have been even fifteen years after the games were being held; a comparatively short time-span from a historical perspective. This is a city subjected to constant architectural, societal and political changes.

4   A Historical Shadow Play

Cunillé's, "mapa d'ombres" relates to the recent history of Catalonia and what has been called a "shadowy city" [of Barcelona] "[u]nder the Franco regime,"[15] and to the gradually unveiled secrets of the protagonists. The title mainly hints to the many social, spatial and historical layers that dwell at the surface of Barcelona's current condition and that make up a complex Catalan capital. In more concrete terms, behind the smooth façade of postmodern Barcelona are years of historical turmoil[16] that in today's global context may seem to have been relegated to the corners of oblivion. However, the opening sequences of the film and its many references to the past assure us that this is far from the case. Thus, in reality, neither Pons nor his protagonists lead lives unaffected by the pre-global era. To quote Gabriela Bruno, "[t]he (im)mobile film spectator" [and the protagonists alike] "moves across an imaginary path, traversing multiple sites and times."[17] The film becomes a mosaic where Pons invites us on a both geographical and historical journey back in time, whereupon he brings us almost seamlessly back into the global present.

   The film opens with an archival map serving as a stark reminder of the Catalan cause and the still problematic relationship between Barcelona and Madrid. This is achieved through footage from the decisive moment when Franco forces entered the Catalan capital unopposed in 1939, with General Juan Bautista Sánchez ultimately thanking the citizens of Barcelona for (involuntarily) facilitating the recognition of Franco as sole leader of all of Spain[18]

15   Resina, *Barcelona's Vocation of Modernity: Rise and Decline of an Urban Image* (Stanford, California: Stanford University Press, 2008), 179.

16   In light of this, Josep. M. Muñoz calls *Barcelona un mapa* "una metáfora sobre la devastación del franquismo." "El hombre invisible." La Vanguardia Opinión, viewed 1 March, 2013, http://hemeroteca.cdmae.cat/jspui/bitstream/65324/6616/1/20080111MAE-VAN-I.pdf.

17   Bruno, "Motion and Emotion: Film and the Urban Fabric," In *Cities in Transition: The Moving Image and the Modern Metropolis*, ed. Andrew Webber and Emma Wilson (London: Wallflower Press, 2008), 19.

18   "These are the images of a hungry Barcelona who throws itself to the streets to cheer the entry of Franco's army. In these images resides the key of a splendid film about the permanent defeat," Cambridge Film Festival 12–22 September 2013: *Barcelona (un mapa)* 2007, La Vanguardia, viewed 10 April 2013, http://www.cambridgefilmfestival.org.uk/films/2012/barcelona.

in a historically significant speech directed straight to the Catalan people and which has been audio-visually recorded for the after-world.

In this initial scene, an effective photo effect is achieved when the image of the Franco general addressing his contemporary audience provokes the dual sensation of the cinematic viewer being likewise spoken to in a manner which merges reality and fiction and which conforms to the statement that "[t]he cinematic image is ... in some sense the perfection of photography: superior in its ranges of nuance of colour or black-and-white to video; firmly within the paradoxical regime of presence-yet-absence that can be called the 'photo effect',"[19] similarly described as cinema being "present absence: it says 'This is was'."[20]

The black and white documentary shots depicting crowds gathering for the arrival of the national forces become additionally effective through Pons' close-ups of select spectators. The viewer is lured into believing that the narrative will linger in the past, but Pons soon proves to us that "cities are spaces of transitions"[21] in more than one way: also as archival storage places that contain architectural pieces of evidence of the past through classical buildings that still remain in the modern city. Through fluid camera movements, the focus on the human element in this emotionally charged urban scene is gradually replaced by a shift into real time, through an establishing shot featuring a now colour-tinged Barcelona skyline. The visual narrative suddenly anchored in the global present perfectly conforms to a "typical exposition of spatial relationships," which

> will begin with an establishing shot of a general location, for example, a cityscape, and might be followed by a shot of a street or building, before moving to an interior shot of an apartment.[22]

Barcelona (un mapa) is, indeed, soon transported into internal milieus and the narrative incorporates conversations between six characters, some of whom

19   John Ellis, *Visible Fictions: Cinema, Television, Video* (London, Boston, Melbourne and Henley: Routledge and Kegan Paul, 1982), 38 and 59.

20   Pons' cinematic portrayal of a *now* and a *then* in this opening scene creates a Barthian photo effect on the viewer, in the sense that images are conjured "of individuals who are apparently present but actually absent." Catherine Elwes, *Video Art: A Guided Tour* (London and New York: I.B. Tauris, 2005), 123.

21   Bruno, "Motion and Emotion: Film and the Urban Fabric," In *Cities in Transition: The Moving Image and the Modern Metropolis*, eds. Andrew Webber and Emma Wilson (London: Wallflower Press, 2008), 18.

22   Barry Jordan and Mark Allinson, *Spanish Cinema: A Student's Guide* (London: Hodder Arnold, 2005), 55.

feature more than once. Regular flashbacks, of e.g. images from within the Liceu Opera House heavy in nostalgia, help continuously interconnect the past and the present. These flashbacks can again be interpreted through a Deleuzian lens as they serve as "'mnemosigns' of flashback memories" that "point toward unorthodox forms of time – a bifurcating time in the flashback, a floating time in dream sequences ..."[23] Literally over in a flash, these brief images serve to create a fluid notion of time and space, collapsing the boundaries between the two. Pons' flashbacks also heighten and underscore the characters' re-narrated personal recollections. References are made to times gone by[24] and to well-known landmarks making up Barcelona's cityscape. Thus, a crystal effect, which recalls Deleuze's notion of cinematic "time crystals,"[25] and a "continuum" is achieved "that fuses the historical past and the present in perpetual exchange."[26] Pujol further notes that "[t]he movie's historical hopscotch subjugates the characters, who cannot conceive an auspicious exit."[27] Indeed, in the film the characters come across as adrift within their urban existence and seem to have lost their footing in life in general. They are stuck in a circular narrative where they recall the past while at the same time they battle to come to grips with Barcelona of today. The story told thus becomes not only a recollection of the past but in equal measure one of dissatisfaction and malaise in the urban present. As effectively summed up by two characters in the first scene of the movie: "- I don't like looking back," "- [and] I don't like looking forwards."[28]

The cartographic overall layout of the film extends also to the protagonists' own generally unexplored inner territory. Their individual preferences, predilections and secrets have all been revealed to the viewer by the end of a visual narrative that leaves us with a multifaceted image of global Barcelona and some of its citizens. Part of such personal idiosyncrasies is Ramon's tendency

---

23   Bogue, *Deleuze on Cinema* (London and New York: Routledge, 2003), 5–6.

24   Interestingly, Ramon, central to the urban narrative, even dreams of the war: "Lately I dream of the war. The day the war finished, mostly" (with an obvious reference to the Spanish Civil War), to which his tenant cynically retorts: "Wars never finish, Ramon. They just go on one after the other, but don't finish." *Barcelona (un mapa)*, directed by Ventura Pons (Barcelona: Generalitat de Caluny – Institut Català de les Indústries Culturals (ICIC), Els Films de la Rambla S.A., Televisió de Catalunya (TV3), and Televisión Española (TVE), 2007), DVD.

25   – as "refracting, filtering, and reflecting surfaces in which the virtual and the actual are made visible and rendered indiscernible as they pass into one another in circuits of exchange." Bogue, *Deleuze on Cinema* (London and New York: Routledge: 2003), 6.

26   Antón Pujol, "Ventura Pons's *Barcelona (un mapa)*: Trapped in the Crystal," *Studies in Hispanic Cinemas* 6, no. 1 (2009): 65.

27   Ibid., 74.

28   *Barcelona (un mapa)*, 2007.

to cross-dress away from the scrutiny of the human eye. He reveals: "Sometimes at the Opera, I hid and disguised himself. I liked going to the costume storeroom and trying things on. There were all sorts of clothes, from every period. If I'd been discovered, they'd have fired me."[29]

Never taking his crossdressing tendencies to an external space, Ramon engages in such displays within the safety of his own home with his wife as apparently sole witness. When at one stage he realises a female tenant has indeed become an unsuspecting second witness, Ramon explains his gender performativity by declaring: "When you dress up, it's like being someone else. As if the costume gave you something you are not ... I do it at home, just for me."[30]

Thus, the film operates on different levels and yet the various narratives are symbolically intertwined. Not only does Ramon – unable to wholly embrace a global present but similarly abhorred by recollections of a belligerent past – seemingly prefer crossdressing as a way to flee into a new, perhaps third reality. But also, crossdressing as a theme in the film correlates with Pons' narrative criss-crossing between different time periods (again cinematographically achieved through real footage versus images of a reconstructed reality).

5   Conclusion

The map of shadows that initially defined Pons' urban map is eventually illuminated in several ways and the shadows from both past and present have largely disappeared by the final scene. The episodic and circular plot development hence comes full circle and any lose ends are tied up. The narrative circularity of the highly postmodern storyline allows us to again witness the same elderly landlords around whom the plot revolves, at the end of the film after having been initially introduced to us in the very first real (fictive) scene. However, their conversation has now taken on a rather different aspect. No longer do they play the formal role of lessors but, rather, they embrace their own peculiarities by voicing secrets in the open; secrets that not even a lengthy marriage has managed to unveil. As they embark on a mutual cross-dressing session in a scene showing Rosa dressed as a man in suit and tie, Ramon only dons lipstick but in doing so he, too, again embraces the mask of performativity. A number of secrets between the two unravel from here, including such varied themes as incest and adultery, and Ramon's confessed burning of the

---

29   Ibid.
30   Ibid.

Liceu Opera House through a sheer act of willpower. As part of this last marital confession the viewer is presented images of a city guidebook that come to life when we follow Ramon's re-narrated walk on foot through the city, through detailed, interactive maps illustrating his urban trajectory. The shadows defining this "gran mapa de sombras"[31] are, through the spouses' mutual confessions as they cross-dress at ease inside their urban apartment, finally gone. And although at the end the viewer is re-introduced to the initial black and white 1939 footage where we realise that the young girl we had seen forming part of the masses is, in fact, Rosa as a girl, Pons eventually proves to us that "[s]iding with the underdogs and opposing the brutality of force is the opposite of fascism. The map of shadows needs not exist anymore."[32]

Although the filmmaker stays clear of anti-Francoist commentaries, his initial – and final – images speak for themselves. What has made the screened urban exposé so effective is Pons' tireless fusion of past and present, reality and fiction which, all in all, resembles postmodern reality where the past is never quite relegated to the past. Rather, "history is a palimpsest, and culture is permeable to time past, time present, and time future."[33]

Bibliography

Barcelona (un mapa). DVD. Directed by Ventura Pons. Barcelona: Generalitat de Catalunya – Institut Català de les Indústries Culturals (ICIC), Els Films de la Rambla S.A., Televisió de Catalunya (TV3), and Televisión Española (TVE), 2007.

Bogue, Ronald. *Deleuze on Cinema*. London and New York: Routledge, 2003.

Bruno, Giuliana. "Site-seeing: Architecture and the Moving Image." *Wide Angle* 19.4 (1997): 8–24.

Bruno, Giuliana. "Motion and Emotion: Film and the Urban Fabric." In *Cities in Transition: The Moving Image and the Modern Metropolis*, edited by Andrew Webber and Emma Wilson, 14–28. London: Wallflower Press, 2008.

Chaudhuri, Shohini. *Contemporary World Cinema: Europe, The Middle East, East Asia and South Asia*. Edinburgh: Edinburgh University Press, 2005.

Ellis, John. *Visible Fictions: Cinema, Television, Video*. London, Boston, Melbourne and Henley: Routledge and Kegan Paul, 1982.

---

31   Ibid.
32   "Barcelona (un mapa) Barcelona (A Map), Spain, 2007," Andy's Film World, viewed 27 February 2013, www.andysfilmworld.blogspot.com.au.
33   Ihab Hassan, *The Postmodern Turn: Essays in Postmodern Theory and Culture* (Ohio: Ohio State University Press, 1987), 88.

Elwes, Catherine. *Video Art: A Guided Tour*. London and New York: I.B. Tauris, 2005.

Harvey, David. *The Condition of Postmodernity: An Enquiry into the Origins of Cultural Change*. Oxford, England, and Cambridge, Massachusetts: Blackwell, 1989.

Hassan, Ihab. *The Postmodern Turn: Essays in Postmodern Theory and Culture*. Ohio: Ohio State University Press, 1987.

Hayward, Susan. *Cinema Studies: The Key Concepts*. London and New York: Routledge, 2000 (second edition).

Jordan, Barry and Mark Allinson. *Spanish Cinema: A Student's Guide*. London: Hodder Arnold, 2005.

Mackay, David. *Modern Architecture in Barcelona (1854–1939)*. UK: The University of Sheffield Printing Unit, 1985.

Martí-Olivella, Jaume. "Catalan Cinema: An Uncanny Transnational Performance." In *A Companion to Catalan Culture*, edited by Dominic Keown, 185–205. Woodbridge, Suffolk: Tamesis, 2011.

Pujol, Antón. "Ventura Pons's *Barcelona (un mapa)*: Trapped in the Crystal." *Studies in Hispanic Cinemas* 6, no. 1 (2009): 65–76.

Resina, Joan Ramon. *Barcelona's Vocation of Modernity: Rise and Decline of an Urban Image*. Stanford, California: Stanford University Press, 2008.

Sánchez, Antonio. "Barcelona's Magic Mirror: Narcissism or the Rediscovery of Public Space and Collective Identity?." In *Constructing Identity in Contemporary Spain. Theoretical Debates and Cultural Practice*, edited by Jo Labanyi, 294–310. Oxford, and New York: Oxford University Press, 2002.

Sorfa, David. "Architorture: Jan Švankmajer and Surrealist Film." In *Screening the City*, edited by Mark Shiel and Tony Fitzmaurice, 100–111. London and New York: Verso, 2003.

Terry, Arthur. "Catalan Literary *Modernisme* and *Noucentisme*: From Dissidence to Order." In *Spanish Cultural Studies. An Introduction. The Struggle for Modernity*, edited by Helene Graham and Jo Labanyi, 55–57. New York: Oxford University Press, 1995.

CHAPTER 12

Developing Patient Oriented Design Criteria for CMHCs in Turkey

Emine Gorgul, Nilay Unsal Gulmez and Ayse Imre Ozgen

1 Background Motives and History of Mental Health Treatments

1.1 Mental Health Treatment in Anatolia

From the 14th century BC to the 4th century AC, health temples named "*Asklepion*" on both sides of the Aegean Sea functioned as the hospitals of the epoch and the priest-doctors applied treatments for both physical maladies and patients with mental illnesses by using methods such as hypnosis and suggestion therapies. (Taneli, 2009). Subsequently, medical centres named "*darussifa*," which were founded during the Great Seljuk Empire were developed in the following epochs of Anatolian Seljuks, while traditional madrasahs were also transformed into healing and recovery houses in those times, in addition to their education facilities (Heybeli, 2009). Those medical centres – *darussifa* – could be defined as general hospitals where all kinds of patients with different diseases, yet every citizen – women, men, children, elderly – were cured without any discrimination for gender, age, ethnicity, religion or race. During those times, *darussifas* were financially supported by the *waqfs*, so that all the services were given for free (Yıldırım, 2010). Since "insanity" was also accepted as a curable disease in the Ottoman Empire, it is known that treatments devoted to mental patients were also taking place in *darussifas* (IBB, 2009).

From the 19th century onwards, accompanying the economic crisis in the Ottoman Empire, *darussifas* were abandoned one by one, while they mostly transformed into mental hospitals named "*bimarhane*" that were sheltering solely homeless people and patients with mental illnesses (Sarı, 2008). For instance, Topbasi Bimarhanesi in Istanbul, which was founded in 1873 within the structure of Atik Valide Complex (Kulliye) was relocated gradually into Resadiye barracks between 1924–29, under the influence of Prof. Dr. Mazhar Osman, the legendary figure in the development of modern Turkish psychiatric hospitals. This hospital still serves in the present day as the "Bakırkoy Prof. Dr. Mazhar Osman Mental Health and Neurological Diseases Education and Research Hospital" (Erkoc et al., 2010). Another *bimarhane* that has reached the present day is Manisa Bimarhanesi in Manisa, one of the important

Anatolian cities, which was founded in 1539 inside the Hafza Sultan Complex (Kulliye). The dilapidated hospital building was relocated after the foundation of the Turkish Republic, to the region where the "Manisa Mental Health and Neurological Diseases Hospital" serves today (TCSB, 2015). Apart from these two hospitals that have survived from the Ottoman times until today, there are seven more remarkable Mental and Neurological Diseases Hospitals (MNDH) founded during the Republican Period in Turkey: Elazig MNDH (1925), Samsun MNDH (1971), Erenkoy MNDH (1976), Adana MNDH (1984), Atakoy MNDH (Trabzon-2003), Bolu Izzet Baysal MNDH (2007) and Tokat MNDH (2013) (TRHastane, 2016).

1.2   Development of Community-Based Mental Health Centres
It is acknowledged that mental health service models in the world are divided into three categories; (1) community-based, (2) hospital-based and (3) community-hospital balance model (TCSB, 2011). The World Health Organization (WHO) emphasizes the significant benefits of adopting the community-based model in favour of human rights (WHO, 2001). In this respect, when mental health services are examined in Turkey it is observed that the hospital-based approach still indicates the highest frequency. The hospital-based approach is fundamentally known as the system where patients are kept in the hospitals during attacks and receive the necessary medication before they are discharged from the hospital. On the other hand, in the community-based model, instead of keeping patients in the psychiatric hospitals for long terms; not only medical, but also social, economic and judicial dimensions of the rehabilitation process are envisioned for curing and preventing the attacks (TCSB, 2011). The "National Mental Health Action Plan" published in 2011 states that for ongoing serious mental diseases, Turkey is obliged to leave the hospital-based approach and move towards a community-based model; in the first place as an intermediary model, the community-hospital balance model will be enacted.

In this respect, Community Mental Health Centres (CMHCs) play a significant role in the transition to the community-based model. The target groups of CMHCs are patients with serious mental disorders – such as schizophrenia and similar psychotic disorders, bipolar affective disorders, etc. – in fact whom had been treated in hospitals during the attacks and were discharged afterwards. CMHCs aim at registering those patients, making daily visits to the patients that cannot reach or access the centre, while trying to support and integrate them into society with various occupational therapies. These therapies are sought to assist individuals' development of motor skills in daily life, whilst offering professional training courses (TCSB, 2014). Moreover, CMHCs also seek to support and educate patients' relatives. In the case of Istanbul, until April

2016 twenty CMHCs operated around major districts of the city, such as Zeytinburnu, Bakırkoy, Esenler, Bahcelievler, Gungoren, Nisantasi, Eyup, Esenyurt, Baggcılar, Kucukcekmece, Fatih, Sarıyer, Kartal, Beylerbeyi, Beykoz, Cekmekoy, Maltepe, Sultanbeyli, Tuzla ve Pendik and the preparations for new ones are in progress.

1.3   Mental Health Approaches from Abroad

Today, very successful examples of community-based approach implementations are observed in European countries. When we look at the history of mental health services and approaches to patients with mental diseases in Europe, we observe that the influence of the Medieval era lasted until the 18th century. Patients were suppressed and excluded from society and also humiliated, while they were imprisoned in hospitals in terrible conditions and were destined to death. Only towards the end of the 18th century, novel practices that would lead the way for modern approaches such as healing spatial conditions, and respect patients' privacy rights were initiated (Almeida et al., 2015).

The history of the modern mental health service approach can be examined in three periods. During the first period between the 19th century and the 20th century, mental health services were hospital-based and were institutionally practiced in huge asylums (Shorter, 2007). In the second period between the Second World War and the 1970's, even though asylums continued to exist, Shorter (2007) stresses that such institutions got worse due to economic difficulties and an increasing number of patients. Nevertheless, the discovery and use of psychosomatic medication and electroshock therapy enabled better control of patients in the 1950's and 1960's, while shifting the socio-political conjuncture of the period that demanded more egalitarian and non-discriminative methods further manifesting the necessity for improving the mental health services and providing more humane (healing) conditions for patients with mental diseases (Piccinelli et al., 2002). It is agreed that the most significant step in the enhancement of mental health services has been the transition from a hospital-based mental health service to a community-based mental health service (Almeida and Killaspy, 2011). The community-based service has been evaluated as essential and more successful in terms of accessibility, sustainability of the treatment and therapies of the patients, as well as support provided to patients' relatives. In this respect, both the development and implementation of education and rehabilitation programs for the adaptability and integration of patients to society, pave the way for satisfactory results for all parties, in favour of human rights and fighting against stigmatization (Almeida et al., 2015). Finally, in the last period from the 1970's until today it is possible to claim that the transition efforts from a hospital-based approach to a community-based approach have

accelerated. So, within this time frame, we witness efforts for meeting requirements of the community-based approach such as abandoning the institutional
structure, closing down the existing Mental and Neurological Disease Hospitals or minimizing their facilities (Table 12.1), transferring patients in need of
immediate medical treatment to psychiatric services of general hospitals, the
foundation of CMHCs, provision of transitional housing, and organizing teams
for home visits of mental patients (Almeida and Killaspy, 2011; Almeida et al.,
2015). Hitherto, the most successful practices of the community-based mental
health approach are observed in Europe; Italy, the UK, Denmark and Holland
especially after the 1960's (Knapp et al., 2007).

2   Research Content, Reasons, Aims and Objectives of the Study

WHO has been encouraging its member states for a while, to increase the level
of attention about mental health, whilst steering them to take further political

TABLE 1   Transfiguring patient number in Psychiatric Hospitals per 100,000 people
between 1998–2012 in Europe

Country Name		Psychiatric Hospitals bed number/100.000 people		
		1998	2008	2012
Austria		33.8	28.5	–
Bulgaria		83.5	–	36.1
Estonia		85.1	–	–
Hungary		–	–	2.8
Ireland		107.2	35.4	21.4
Italy	Emilia-Romagna	0	0	0
	Lazio	0	0	0
	Lombardia	11.2	0	0
	Veneto	0	0	0
Portugal		21	13	10
Spain		43	37	25
The UK		-	14	–

SOURCE: ALMEIDA ET AL., 2015.

measures and to develop related plans (WHO, 2011). In accordance with these calls improvement and implementations, Turkey initiated its "National Mental Healthcare Action Plan" in 2011 that will be further applicable until 2023 (Yılmaz, 2012). This action plan strongly defends the necessity for a shift from old-fashioned hospital-based treatments that heal permanent heavy mental diseases, into community-centred treatment methodologies. This novel approach offers a transitional model, entitled "community-hospital balance model" as an initial step in this transformation process. Accordingly, in 2011 "Community Mental Healthcare Centres (CMHC) Regulations" were launched, and were revised in 2014 (TCSB, 2011).

When CMHC Regulations are examined in detail, it is observed that they are broadly missing architectural and interior architectural essences in terms of spatial configuration and comfort. Particularly, when Act 6 in Section II entitled "Physical Conditions, Tools and Equipment Standards" is examined, it is observed that most of the definitions relating to CMHC spaces are poorly defined, even without indicating any program requirements or specific spatial features. Moreover, it is also revealed that the physical and spatial requirements are mostly not mentioned. For instance, the act begins like roughly stating the location of CHMCs such as "preferably located in a central area, easily accessible by public transportations, and as a closed space at least having a 300 m2 footprint, accommodating group therapy spaces, etc." (TCSB, 2014). Hence, it is possible to assert that CMHC regulations remain inadequate in terms of constituting the spatial context and related infrastructure. Departing from these fundamental deficiencies in the CMHC regulations, this initial research was executed in terms of focusing on the healing capacities of spaces and the immense importance of the spatial qualities on behalf of creating positive sensorial impact, not only on the psyche of the mentally disordered patients, their families and the staff, but also their efficiency in healing process and work environment. In other words, this research offers a comprehensive revision of current CMHC regulations in the scope of these mentioned spatial relations while seeking to generate a design manual as its major objective, so that it holistically introduces the CMHC design criteria both for the designers and for the upcoming implementations. In this respect, a detailed survey and research was conducted in collaboration with the ENPH-Erenkoy Neuro Psychiatric Hospital in Istanbul, and its three branching CMHC units in Beylerbeyi, Sultanbeyli and Cekmekoy districts were selected as case studies in the field research. Thus, the physical and spatial requirements of the CMHCs were examined from diverse approaches according to both different user profiles (patients, healthcare staff-doctors-nurses, etc., patient families) and spatial qualities (spatial configuration, components of interior space and comfort conditions, as well as furniture and equipment).

3   Research Approach and Methodology

Since there has been an immense absence of any resources about recently
emerging CMCHs in Turkey, as well as the lack of any hypothetical and empirical feedback about the ongoing implementations given; this research focuses
on developing relevant assets and the initial inventory in the field, while contributing to the literature in the discipline by sharing the knowledge gathered
from on-site analysis. Thus, also referring to the growing importance of Evidence Based Design in healthcare design, the EBD methodology has been deployed as the essential strategy for this research to attain first-hand data from
the CMHC users, in order to obtain the relevant information and to generate an
appropriate reference to the discipline.

   So, as a comprehensive design strategy EBD covers various tactics to attain
the projected goals. For instance, extensive literature reviews, a detailed analysis of the existing projects and examples, case studies and surveys on site,
various experiments and observations for gathering the relevant data, assert-
ing and narrowing down the findings into applicable interim-outputs for the
design decisions, and finally generating the optimum design project are the
consequent steps of the EBD methodology that are also deployed in this research (McCullough, 2010). In this regard, while deploying EBD as the essential
strategy for the research, a mixed model of both quantitative and qualitative
methods has been utilized in various steps of the research process to attain the
goals and the objectives. The four consequent steps of the research process are
outlined as follows:

1.   Initially an extensive literature review was conducted to mark the inter-
       national studies and to map the progress in the field.
2.   In the second step, the existing conditions in the CMHCs were examined
       through three selected cases. This examination process systematically
       enfolds four sub-phases of quantitative and qualitative research.
   2a.   Quantitative values of both user numbers and spatial dimensions
          have been gathered.
   2b.   2011 and 2014 dated "Community Mental Healthcare Centres
          (CMHC) Regulations" were examined in detail. Consequently, ini-
          tial observations about the existing cases were cross-read with the
          mentioned regulations, in order to evaluate the relevancy between
          legislative frame and current implementations.
   2c.   After basic – quantitative – on site observations about the physical
          spaces of the three cases; qualitative examinations have been car-
          ried out. In this regard, departing from the importance of user expe-
          rience in the design processes semi-structured intensive interviews

were held in each CMHC unit, to reveal the psychic and physical influences of the spatial setup on the users. The CMCH users have been divided into to three categories; patients, healthcare staff (physiatrists, psychologists, social-service specialists, nurses and other officers) and finally patient families.

2d.   During the semi-structured intensive interviews with the sample group, a questionnaire consisting of open-ended questions has been deployed, and voice recording has been used in each meeting. The interview questions focus on three major categories of the CMHC spaces, such as spatial configuration; interior space comfort conditions; as well as furniture and equipment.

3.   In the third step, analysis of the quantitative and qualitative data as well as the assessment of the initial findings were evaluated. In this regard, in terms of quantitative research, numeric analysis and comparisons between the numbers of users (patients, staff and patient families) and again dimensional analysis and assessment of physical space were done. On the other hand, in terms of qualitative research, a content analysis method was deployed to analyse the data gathered from the interviews.

4.   In the final step, in light of findings from the quantitative and content analysis, building program requirements and design criteria as well as the CMHC design manual have been put forth as a reference for the upcoming constructions of the CMHC units as well as the remodelling and upgrading of the existing spaces.

4   Findings and Concluding Remarks

Being essential components of public health system, CMHC units ought to be implemented in respect of specific design criteria. Although the Turkish Ministry of Health generated a directive for the constitution of CMHC units, and enacted it in 2011 and revised in 2014, it is observed that this directive does not specify minimum requirements in detail. Moreover, a rapid investigation of the existing CMHCs around the Istanbul region reveals that those centres are mostly placed in residential apartments, that are far from meeting the requirements of the deficient directive (Table 12.2).

The findings of the qualitative part of this inquiry and related interviews approve the main argument of this research, which states that the design criteria of CMHCs have a deeper impact on the psychology and efficiency of patients, patient families and health personnel, directly related with the benefit that they

TABLE 2   Comparison of CMHC codes and regulation through the cases.

	CMHC Regulations (06.03.2014)Section 2/Act 6	Beylerbeyi CMHC	Sultanbeyli CMHC	Cekmekoy TRSM
Physical Conditions	At least 300 m² footprint	X	X	X
	Individual/detached building	X	X	X
	Located on the ground floor or connected floor	✓	X	X
	Easily accessible by public transportation	✓	✓	✓
	Central location	X	X	✓
	Proper deployment of fire safety regulations	X	X	X
Building	Entrance area	✓	✓	X
Programme	Welcome and check-in counter, security, waiting area, information and orientation boards, seating areas..	✓	✓	✓
	Group therapy room	✓	✓	✓
	Adequate number of tables and chairs, and a lecture board, enough space for meetings and internal education sessions.	✓	✓	X
	Hobby and rehabilitation room	✓	✓	X
	Room should be of an adequate size, have the right dimensions and accommodate the adequate number of sinks, tables, chairs/stools, exhibition shelves, boards, and lockers.	X	X	X
	Library and reading room	X	X	X
	Room should be of an adequate size, have the right dimensions and accommodate the adequate number of tables, chairs, boards, computers and bookcases for reading and internet access facilities.	X	X	X

Criterion			
Mensa / Kitchen	✓	✓	✓
Room should be of an adequate size and have the right dimensions to accommodate the facilities of cooking and food service for patients and staff.	✓	✓	✓
Therapy kitchen	X	X	X
Room should be of an adequate size, have the right dimensions and accommodate the adequate amount of furniture and equipment for the volunteers both from public and from patient families, as well as patients that are willing to serve as cooks as the part of healing therapies.	X	X	X
Multi-purpose room	✓	✓	✓
A room for the patients to rest and sit, should accommodate enough equipment.	X	X	X
Treatment and examination room	✓	✓	✓
Room should be of an adequate size, have the right dimensions and accommodate the adequate amount of furniture and equipment for injection and any examination cases.	✓	✓	✓
Sports area	X	X	X
Adequate ventilation, shower facilities and changing rooms if located indoors.	X	X	X
Consultation room	✓	✓	✓
Individual locked cupboards, table, chair, computer, and folder storage.	✓	✓	✓

TABLE 2   Comparison of CMHC codes and regulation through the cases (*cont.*)

CMHC Regulations (06.03.2014)Section 2/Act 6	Beylerbeyi CMHC	Sultanbeyli CMHC	Cekmekoy TRSM
Team study room (archive)	X	X	X
Accommodates the adequate amount of furniture and equipment for archiving folders and records, computers, etc.	X	X	X
Cleaning materials and equipment storage	X	X	X
Toilets	X	X	✓
Accommodates the adequate number of cubical for patient and personnel, women and men. Segregation is essential, doors should swing to the corridor, sink and closet should be inserted.	✓	✓	✓
Accessible toilets	X	X	✓
There should be at least one cubicle.	X	X	✓

get from these centres. Even though CMHCs are very important in terms of the transition from a hospital-based model to a community-based model, in the initial cases they are obliged to fit into places; mostly apartments addressed by the municipalities. Thus, due to insufficient conditions, building programs could not respond the requirements adequately, so that the current CMHCs still remain as successors of the hospitals. It is believed that this situation retards and even constitutes an impediment in terms of reaching the goals of CMHCs.

In light of qualitative and quantitative research on the site, essential program requirements for the spatial configuration of CMHC units can be listed as follows:
– Consulting rooms in accordance with the number of consultants
– Expert doctor rooms in accordance with the number of expert doctors
– Minimum one treatment room
– Kitchen
– Therapy kitchen
– Minimum two rooms for occupational therapy
– Music room
– Sports area
– A minimum of four toilets allocated for patients/personnel and women/ men (one of which should be designed according to universal design principles)
– Staff lounge
– Archive
– Lounge and television room
– Cafeteria/eating area
– Entrance-secretary/registration- waiting area

Yet, in relation to the spatial program requirements, major themes that emerge as significant design issues in CMHC units both in program standards and in user interaction can be elaborated into fourteen subcases:
1. Location and Transportation: CMHCs are to be located in the central areas that are easily reached and accessible by public transportation.
2. Garden: Each CMHC is to be located in a garden plot, where seating, outdoor sports areas, and hobby gardens for the patients' therapies and use are located within this garden space.
3. Dimensions: CMHC spaces are to be designed by offering enough spatial qualities for its users where they can move and work comfortably, while maintaining spacious and comfortable environments that also retain the social space dimensions. Besides, in accordance with the earlier 2011 "Community Mental Healthcare Centres (CMHC) Regulations," at least 300 m² footprint rule does apply to the CMHCs.

4.   Spatial Qualifications: CMHCs are to be located in individual or detached buildings that have modest architectural characteristics, and are always well-maintained; preferably have a view, and possess home-like indoor atmospheres that may not cause any subliminal hints about psychiatric hospitals.

5.   Activities: In order to answer to the varying demands of the patients, CMHCs are to be designed by offering at least three different therapeutic activities such as, group therapy, arts therapy and music activity, that all having a dedicated space for each.

6.   Spatial Configuration: In addition to the fundamental spaces that are mentioned in the building program requirements, spaces like smoking rooms and cafeterias are also to be located in CMHCs. However, due to the functional hierarchy and privacy, consulting and therapy rooms are to be designed farther from the heavy circulation of the entrance, waiting room and hobby spaces.

7.   Materials: In favour of security and comfort conditions, it is recommended that non-inflammable, non-slippery, easy-clean surfaces and materials are chosen in the CMHC spaces. In addition, to maintain the patients' comfort, softer finishing is recommended on seating elements (yet avoiding selection of super soft materials).

8.   Colors: During the color selection of interior surfaces, deployment of extra-stimulant colors are to be avoided, while light and pastel tones are recommended. In addition, in order to break the monotone configuration and similarities between the spaces, different colors may be applied on the interior surfaces.

9.   Lighting: CMHC spaces are to be designed to get the maximum benefit of the day light. When natural light is not sufficient, an adequate amount of lighting should be provided through artificial light sources. As an artificial light source, diffuse chartered elements of ceiling armatures (not floor lamps nor hanging elements) with daylight colors are recommended.

10.   HVAC: Central HVAC systems are recommended in the CMHCs.

11.   Sound Control: In order to attain privacy and sound comfort conditions in the consulting rooms as well as within the whole CMHC environment, doors, windows and partition elements with sound insulation layers should be chosen.

12.   Furniture: Furniture inside the CMHC units should be ergonomic, comfortable, durable and functional. The furniture sets within the rooms should respond to the needs of the assigned functions of the spaces and should be in accordance with each other, as varying elements of the same

furniture series. Also, in order to strengthen the feeling of "home" and individualization of the space, furniture and accessories such as armchairs, carpets, framed pictures and paintings, as well as vases may be used within the spaces.

13.   Seating Elements: Adequate number of mobile seating elements with enough comfort performance should be provided for the users. Also, the same type of furniture is recommended for both patient and staff in order to keep the equivalency and trust between the parties.

14.   Security: There should be at least one qualified and inter-service trained security personnel in every CMHC unit. Besides, it is also quite important to employ the security personal with civil outfits, not wearing a uniform to offend the patients. On the other hand, again for the same reasons, the spatial precautions should be indirect, hidden and obscure such as partially open window wings, unbreakable windows, etc.

As a result, it is observed that, in order to succeed in the shift from hospital-based treatments into community-centred mental healthcare services, rapid implementations and actions are launched in Turkey. The increasing number of active CMHCs from seven (7) at the beginning of this research proposal to twenty (20) at the end of the research project also approve this acceleration. The growing numbers also highlight the importance that has been given to the mental healthcare services in Turkey. It is believed that this research that offers an initial design manual for CMHC spaces, would pave the way for positive progress of Turkey's mental healthcare services in the near future.

Acknowledgements

We would like to extend our thanks to TUBITAK – The National Scientific and Research Council of Turkey – for the funding support, and NPH-Erenkoy Neuro Psychiatric Hospital psychiatrists Dr. Haluk Usta and Assoc. Prof. Dr. Huseyin Gulec for their collaboration and support throughout the field research.

Bibliography

Caldas de Almeida, J. M., and Helen Killaspy. *Long-term Mental Healthcare for People with Severe Mental Disorders*. Europe Union Reports, 2011.

Caldas de Almeida, J. M., Pedro Mateus, and Gina Tomé. *Joint Action on Mental Health and Well-being Towards Community-Based and Socially Inclusive Mental Health Care*. Europe Union Reports, 2015.

Erkoc, Sahap, Fulya Kardes, and Fatih Artvinli. "Bakirkoy Prof. Dr. Mazhar Osman Ruh Sagligi ve Sinir Hastalıkları Egitim ve Arastırma Hastanesi'nin Kısa Tarihi." *Dusunen Adam Psikiyatri ve Norolojik Bilimler Dergisi* 25 (2010): 1–12.

Heybeli, Nurettin. "Sultan Bayezid II Külliyesi: One of the Earliest Medical Schools Founded in 1488." *Clinical Orthopaedics and Related Research* 467 (2009): 2457–2463.

İstanbul Sifahaneleri. Istanbul: IBB- İstanbul Buyuksehir Belediyesi, 2009.

Knapp, Martin, David McDaid, Elias Mossialos, and Graham Thornicroft. *Mental Health Policy and Practice Across Europe.* Glasgow: McGraw-Hill Open University Press, 2007.

McCullough, Cynthia S. *Evidence-Based Design for Healthcare Facilities.* Illinois: Tau International, 2010.

Piccinelli, Marco, Pierluigi Politi, and Francesco Barale. "Focus on Psychiatry in Italy." *British Journal of Psychiatry* 181 (2002): 538–544.

Sari, Nil, and Burhan Akgun, "Turk Tarihinde Psikiyatriye Bakıs." *I.U. Cerrahpasa Tip Fakultesi Surekli Tıp Egitimi Etkinlikleri, Turkiye'de Sik Karsilasilan Psikiyatrik Hastaliklar Sempozyum Dizisi* 62 (2008): 1–24.

Shorter, Edward. "The Historical Development of Mental Health Services in Europe." In *Mental Health Policy and Practice Across Europe*, edited by Martin Knapp, David McDaid, Elias Mossialos, and Graham Thornicroft, 15–33. Glasgow: McGraw-Hill Open University Press, 2007.

Taneli, Baha. "Cumhuriyet'ten Once ve Sonra Ulkemizde Saglik Kurumları ve Cocuk Hastaneleri." *Ege Pediatri Bülteni* 16–2 (2009): 95–110.

TCSB (Turkiye Cumhuriyeti Saglik Bakanligi). *Ulusal Ruh Sagligi Eylem Plani 2011–2023.* Ankara: TCSB, 2011.

TCSB (Turkiye Cumhuriyeti Saglik Bakanligi). *Toplum Ruh Sagligi Merkezleri Hakkinda Yonerge.* Ankara: TCSB, 2014.

TCSB. *TCSB Manisa Ruh Sagligi ve Hastalikları Hastanesi.* Ankara: TCSB, 2015.

TRHastane. Devlet Ozel Saglik Kurumlari Rehberi. TRHastane: 2016.

WHO (World Health Organization). *Mental Health: New Understanding, New Hope.* Geneva: WHO, 2001.

WHO (World Health Organization). *Mental Health Atlas 2011.* Geneva: WHO, 2011.

Yıldırım, Nuran. *Istanbul'un Saglik Tarihi.* Istanbul: Istanbul Universitesi, 2010.

Yılmaz, Volkan. "Ruh Sagligi Politikaları: Tespitler ve Oneriler, 3–4." *RUSIHAK* (April 2012).

Index of Names

Index of Terms and Concepts

Printed in the United States
By Bookmasters